MW01098678

BALANCE:

The Wellness
and Weight-Control Primer
for Men

R.M. Jensen

R & E Publishers

R&E Publishers
P.O. Box 2008, Saratoga, CA 95070
Tel: (408) 866-6303   Fax: (408) 866-0825

Book Design and Typesetting by **elletro** Productions

Cover Design by R.M. Jensen
Cover Art by Kaye Quinn

ISBN 1-56875-065-X

Library of Congrss Cataloging-in-Publication Data
Jensen, R.M.
    Balance: the wellness and weight-control primer for men / R.M. Jensen.
        p. cm
    ISBN 1-56875-065-X : $11.95
1. Reducing. 2. Men--Health and hygiene. I. Title. II. Title: Wellness ans weight-control primer for men.
    RM222.2J5   1993
    613'.04234--dc20

                                                              93-28152
                                                              CIP

Designed, typeset and totally manufactured in the
United States of America.

BECOMING A DEDICATED PARTICIPANT
IN THE BALANCE PROGRAM CAN:

═══════════════════════════════

- HELP YOU LEARN SKILLS THAT CAN BE USED FOR SUCCESS IN ALL AREAS OF YOUR LIFE.

- HELP YOU DEVELOP FEELINGS OF ACHIEVEMENT AND SELF ESTEEM THAT WILL ENHANCE THE OVERALL STATE OF YOUR WELLNESS.

- PROVIDE YOU WITH PERSONAL VALUE FULFILLMENT.

═══════════════════════════════

- **BALANCE** IN YOUR FOOD CHOICES AND EATING HABITS

- **BALANCE** IN YOUR PHYSICAL ACTIVITY

- **BALANCE** IN YOUR ATTITUDES AND BEHAVIOR

EQUALS

WELLNESS IN MIND, BODY AND SPIRIT

CONTENTS

VI. PHYSICAL FITNESS

VII. STABILIZATION AND MAINTENANCE

* ACTIVITY WORKSHEETS
(PLEASE PHOTOCOPY AS NECESSARY)

PREFACE

In very general terms, most overweight individuals will fall into one of these three categories:

1. The "conditionally" overweight

Specific circumstances have brought about a weight gain (activities such as stopping smoking, over-indulgence during holiday season or vacation).

2. The "cosmetically" overweight

While they may have been overweight for a long period of time, excess weight has usually been put on in a creeping fashion as age and lack of exercise take their toll. From a medical standpoint, these men may not be obese (defined as more than 20% overweight), but weight loss could improve health, appearance, and vitality.

3. The "chronically" obese

Excess weight is a result of continued long-term over-consumption and/or poor food choices. These individuals have a food addiction and will most probably have been obese for a better part of their adult lives. Their weight problem involves more than just food.

The Balance program can be of help in all three circumstances. It will, however, be of most benefit to those men who are in the chronically overweight category. Learning to understand and change the lifestyle and behavioral aspects that have contributed to their weight problem is a key element in bringing about desired changes.

Many men who need to lose weight may not be motivated to do so until they make the very real connection between obesity and either actual or potential health problems. This motivation can be the result of a heart attack, stroke, or other serious illness — either their own or that of friends or family. In many cases, the realization comes as function of mid-life awareness. Excess weight that in the past was either ignored or considered an aspect of perceived masculinity is now viewed in a new light: as a health hazard. A majority of these men, once they become aware of the reality, are willing and even eager to rid themselves of excess pounds. They do, however, need some specific education and techniques to help them accomplish it.

It is important to understand the reason or combination of reasons behind the specific weight problem. Knowing why you are overweight can help you change habits and behaviors that endanger your health and well-being.

In order to achieve long-term success with a weight-loss program, certain attitudes and actions are necessary:

1. The most important of these is *motivation*. You must genuinely want to lose weight and be willing to try to make the needed changes in eating and thinking patterns in order to succeed. You also need to realize that these changes come about as the result of your own choices, not someone else's inflexible rules.

2. In addition to motivation, you need sufficient eating, nutrition, and exercise *knowledge* to allow you to accomplish your desired weight-loss goal.

3. Armed with motivation and necessary knowledge, you will also need to learn specific *techniques* and *strategies* that can be used to help you achieve and maintain weight reduction.

The information and activities in the Balance program are compiled in workbook fashion that encourages your participation to develop a tailor-made plan. The program is designed to both stimulate and sustain motivation. It is a tool that you can use to become a person without a weight problem.

You will find throughout this workbook that I have used the term "we" rather than "I" because my research and methodology includes ideas and opinions of many individuals with whom I have come in contact. I believe it is important to know that the information and strategies reflect the knowledge and ideas of many who have been successfully involved in weight loss.

I

WHAT THE BALANCE CONCEPT IS ALL ABOUT

WHY A PROGRAM FOR MEN ONLY?

There are several reasons why a weight-loss program for men needs to be different than one used by women.

1. Many men lack food and nutritional knowledge, so they unknowingly make poor eating choices. They are more likely than women to need food education.

2. Many men eat food chosen and prepared by someone else that may include high levels of fat and sugar. If this is your situation, you may have to be in charge of your own meal planning, shopping and cooking.

3. Many men have never been on a weight-loss program, and they need guidance and support to achieve their weight-loss goals.

4. Most participants (up to 80%) in the support groups of weight-loss programs and clinics are women, and men may feel uncomfortable being part of these groups.

5. For many men, it is difficult to communicate the problems and concerns they have related to weight loss. They may only feel at ease with an exclusively male group.

6. Men's bodies are different than women's, so they need food and exercise plans tailored to their special needs.

7. Many men view excess weight as power and need to better understand the health hazards connected with being overweight.

THE BALANCE PROGRAM MEETS THESE NEEDS!

Men view their bodies somewhat differently than women. A woman will be concerned if her clothes don't fit or if she is so overweight that she believes it adversely affects her appearance. A man, on the other hand, may seldom look at his body in a full-length mirror. Except when they shave, many men aren't very conscious of their appearance. They are more likely to view their excess weight as a sign of strength or even virility. They have, in many cases, been programmed by our American culture into equating size with strength—and therefore with masculinity.

Especially as they approach middle age, men may try to hold onto what they believe is a youthful image of "bigness" remembering when they used to play football or wrestle or some other physical sport where they tested their strength and agility against others. This isn't meant to suggest that there is anything wrong with this kind of self image, but rather to demonstrate how that kind of thinking can relate to overeating. In the past, much of the American male's self esteem has been connected to his physical size and strength. Today, however, physical size and strength are being reappraised in terms of physical fitness. Paunchiness and flab are regarded as potential health hazards, and being a "big guy" has taken a back seat to being a "healthy guy!"

What we would like you to consider is reconnecting your self image to a more appropriate image of health and fitness. For most of us the time for team sports that required speed and strength are behind us. What should now be more important is how you feel and how you *will feel* in the coming years.

Because of improved health knowledge and health care, man has increased his potential life span. With a little luck (and a little good care), you should now be able to enjoy a long, active life. A great deal of attention in our society is currently being directed not just to living longer, but also to improving the quality of those extended years.

While our grandfathers may have engaged in hard physical labor on farm or in factory in the past century, most of us now have a much more sedentary lifestyle. We have become a society of technical "knowledge" workers. The trade off, of course, is that with today's abundance of readily available food and the reduction of required physical effort, we are faced with a new health challenge. Do we want to be unhealthy and overweight with the corresponding physical incapacities in our extended years, or would we rather enjoy those extra years with a healthy, active lifestyle? The answer seems obvious. It brings to mind the old saying, "If I had known I was going to live this long, I'd have taken better care of myself."

Well, gentlemen, the good news is that (statistically speaking) you are going to live longer than your ancestors. The bad news is that you may not do it with any degree of quality if you don't start thinking and caring and doing something about it now.

The quality of your future life, especially in your middle and senior years, will be dependent upon what you do right now related to your lifestyle, physical movement, nutrition, attitudes and relationships.

This, then, is the objective of the BALANCE concept: to provide you with information and support directed at your specific needs so you can achieve and maintain the quality of life you deserve!

A NEW WAY OF THINKING

The BALANCE program is not a revolutionary new concept, rather it is a structured program to help develop you a new way of thinking and living. Similar information is available from a variety of sources. However, there doesn't seem to be a singular source combining all the necessary aspects into a program designed just for men. Related to their weight goals, men's motivations differ from those of women. Men also encounter situations and reactions to weight loss that are unique to their sex. To be successful, a weight-loss program needs to address these needs.

Although the concepts and techniques in this book will be useful for anyone trying to lose and keep off excess weight, the workbook has been created primarily for men who are more than 20% overweight and/or men who have a chronic problem with taking weight off and keeping it off. The BALANCE program was developed with the express view that the health and well-being of these men is endangered by their food addiction and resultant obesity, and it offers a system by which they can attain and maintain control over this excess weight that is endangering their wellness.

I encourage those who want to participate in this program to use it in conjunction with any healthy weight-loss food plan of their choice (such as WEIGHT WATCHERS) or to use the food plan that is suggested in this workbook. You may even be interested in starting your own support group which can be formed based upon the concepts presented in the BALANCE program.

Quick-loss weight programs certainly offer emotional appeal, but there is ample evidence that these kinds of programs ultimately don't work. While the desire to eat is instinctive, the kinds of foods and the quantities you eat are more a result of conditioning and habit. Habits can be changed. New, more beneficial ways of eating can be learned; not just for the objective of losing weight, but also for the very important objective of adopting and maintaining a healthy lifestyle. That is where we are directing our efforts with this program: to help you develop new ways of eating that work better for you and that will become a permanent way of life. The critical elements that will aid you in doing this include:

> Your commitment
>
> Behavior and attitude changes, if needed
>
> Following food and water guidelines
>
> Exercise
>
> A support group and/or wellness partner

Obesity wasn't something that happened to you overnight, and you won't get it under control overnight. By learning new attitudes and eating habits, however, you will be able to reduce your weight and become more healthy. Then you must incorporate this new way of thinking and eating into your future lifestyle so you can continue to be a person without a weight problem.

HOW TO USE THIS WORKBOOK

1. Before beginning the BALANCE program, read through the entire workbook. It includes information plus activities related to:

> Health and nutrition
>
> Food and eating
>
> Using the positive power of the mind
>
> Physical fitness
>
> Monitoring your program
>
> Stabilization and maintenance

2. The worksheet activities throughout this workbook are to help you identify the behaviors and attitudes in your life that you would like to change or modify that affect your overeating. (Some you will want to photocopy because you will need to use them more than once.) Suggestions are also given that will help you accomplish these changes. Remember that no one except you will see these activity worksheets, so try to be as honest with yourself as possible. If some worksheets seem not to apply to your particular situation, skip these. If you encounter some mental resistance related to certain activities, leave them for the time being, but try to come back to them later. Also, you may wish to repeat certain worksheets periodically as you feel they will be of benefit to you. You will find that your behavior and your attitudes may change as you progress, and redoing an activity will provide you with a basis of comparison so you can review your progress.

3. While using this system may seem somewhat involved at first, you will quickly become familiar with your routine, and using it will provide both motivation and a structure that will aid you in achieving your goal.

4. While the BALANCE program has attempted to cover all aspects of weight loss in a general fashion, we suggest you also access additional sources if you desire more in-depth information on specific areas of importance to you.

THE BALANCE PROGRAM

You are a special person. There is no other individual who is quite like you. That is why your wellness plan will be one that works for you...because you are designing it to fit your unique needs.

Most diet plans are designed to fit a group mode: one plan for everybody. There is very little individualization within these programs. In other words, you must go on a plan designed by someone else that may have been very successful for them, but may or may not work for you. Many of these plans focus on the body only, ignoring the impact our minds have on our bodies.

Standard diet plans offered through self-help books and traditional diet clinics may not have worked for you in the past because you are used to making your own decisions, not following the dictates of someone else's philosophy. This is the way you operate, and it works for you. That is why the BALANCE program offers a broad scope of information and options. You incorporate your choices and your decisions. The plan must include your participation in its creation in order to ensure your commitment.

The BALANCE program is designed to provide you with a framework, information, motivation, and encouragement that will allow you to accomplish the success you are seeking. It is not per se a weight-loss program. It is not a dieting plan. It is a program to allow you to become a person without a food or weight problem. It is a program that you will help to design so that it will meet your special needs.

Working together, we will structure a customized plan for you, the ultimate objective of which is the accomplishment of the goals you set. The method by which you will achieve your goals will include a process of exploring and using various techniques that you select that involve both your mind and your body.

The processes involved in weight loss are highly complex. Modern-day science is only just beginning to understand the close interrelationship between mind and body. It's not entirely understood, but it is a fact that this interrelationship can be used to your advantage. It is important that a wellness program work for the total you...the you that incorporates your mind, your body, and your spirit. In using the word spirit, we don't wish to imply a particular religious philosophy, but rather to identify that area in each of us that is our awareness ... our individual consciousness.

For many, food represents more than just daily nourishment. We eat not only because we are physically hungry. We eat because we are using food as a reward; we eat as a reason to procrastinate; we eat to reduce the craving for alcohol or cigarettes; we eat as an excuse for why we can't do or have certain things in our life. Many of us were programmed and brainwashed into overeating early in life when we couldn't get down from the table until we had cleaned our plates.

Later, eating became part of our social culture—(Let's go get a hamburger and a milkshake after the game, guys.) Social gatherings were fun for us—and most included food of some kind. Or maybe we went home and ate because we weren't invited to the party.

Our American culture and society are inundated with food. The largest percentage of money spent for TV advertising relates to food. We are one of the few countries that can measure its wealth by its girth. Today, more than 34 million of us are obese (more than 20% overweight). Let's face it — most of us can afford to eat whatever we choose—and we chews a lot, guys! Add to this the fact that between the ages of 25 and 45, your caloric requirements drop by some 10% to 20% and between ages 45 and 65 they drop still another *20%*. Do you begin to see how being overweight is a complex problem with no one simple solution for everyone?

If you have a chronic problem with overweight and overeating, your problem is not about food. If you view the situation from one of cause and effect, food is the effect you are allowing to control your life. The cause is something you will need to spend some time figuring out.

The list of why we overeat is a long one. It is important that you try to define your unique reasons for overeating, and then try to channel the compulsion or addiction or urge that is causing you to be unwell into some more constructive directions. The BALANCE program will show you how this can be done. The rest is up to you.

The list on the following page identifies 14 conditions that are possible contributors to obesity. After you have familiarized yourself with these, complete the activity worksheet that relates to your specific situation. Understanding your individual impacts and triggers will give you a better grasp on how to overcome the weight obstacle with which you are now faced.

CONDITIONS THAT CONTRIBUTE TO OVERWEIGHT

THERE ARE MANY REASONS WHY WE OVEREAT OR ARE OVERWEIGHT:

1. Poor food choices and poor eating habits: (Too much fat and too many refined carbohydrates in our diet.)

2. Parental value system: (The clean plate club, the starving children in China, and using food as a reward or soother.)

3. Inherited genetic structure: (Too many fat cells and a predisposition to obesity.)

4. Long-term psychological problems: (Food as a substitute for self-esteem, as a "Band-Aid" for unexpressed emotions, etc.)

5. Short-term psychological reasons: (Burnout, stress, anxiety, boredom.)

6. Health-related conditions: (Alcoholism, diabetes, hypoglycemia, thyroid malfunction, ulcers, etc.)

7. Societal/lifestyle influence: (Eating as entertainment, holidays, vacations.)

8. Affluent society: (An abundance of food is available, and Americans can afford to overeat.)

9. Physical aging process: (Loss of metabolism from aging and too little physical activity.)

10. Mind set: ("Big" equates with power and strength.)

11. Dysfunctional family background: (Victims of child abuse, or adult children of alcoholics.)

12. Ethnic background: (Heavy, rich foods as a learned eating pattern.)

13. Lack of knowledge of what constitutes a healthy diet.

14. Busy lifestyle that encourages eating fattening, commercially prepared, and "fast" foods.

WHY AM I OVERWEIGHT ACTIVITY

Based upon the information on the preceding page, which influences do I believe have helped bring about my weight problem? (Fill in the boxes)

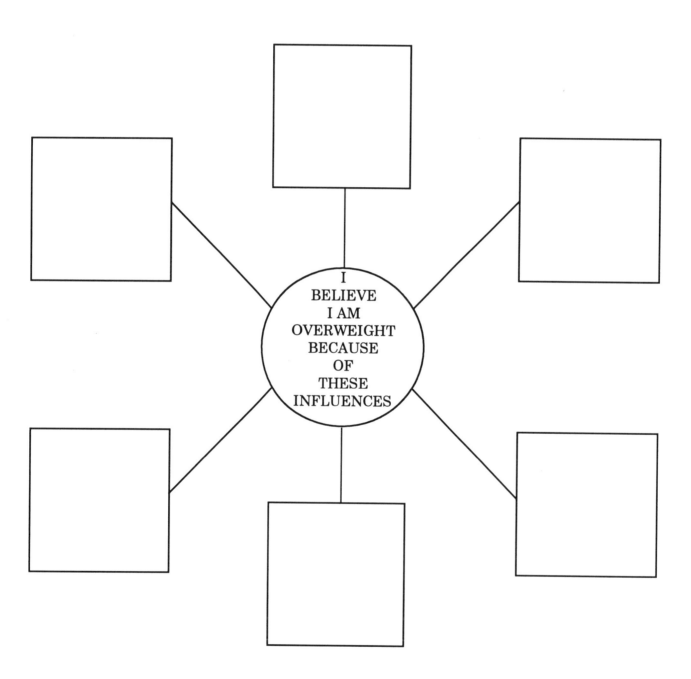

WHO HAS HELPED ME BECOME OVERWEIGHT?

Once you have completed the worksheet where you have identified what you believe are some of the specific causes of your overweight situation, we'd like you to take this additional step. If at first you seem to have some reservations or resistance to doing this activity, leave it for the time being, but please do come back to it later on as you progress with your program.

1. Who do I believe has contributed to my weight or overeating problem in the past?

2. How did they influence me?

3. Who do I believe influences my overeating or weight problem at present?

4. How do they influence my eating behavior?

AFTER YOU COMPLETE THIS ACTIVITY, PLEASE COMPLETE THE FOLLOWING FORGIVENESS WORKSHEET.

FORGIVENESS ACTIVITY

What forgiving means as we intend it to be used in this activity is a letting-go process. It is a means by which you can free yourself of old resentments and old angers. Forgiveness does not mean that you are approving someone else's (or your own) past behavior or actions, just that you no longer want those negative feelings within you. Resentment, jealousy, and similar feelings don't hurt the person you're projecting them against: they hurt you! They cause undesirable stress reactions that can jeopardize your health—not the health of the person you are angry with (unless, of course, that person is you.)

It's important for you to acknowledge that you as well as others may have had some impact on your weight situation, and then to release those feelings. It doesn't really matter whose fault it is that you are overweight (yours or someone else's or both). Get rid of the old feelings! You've got much better things to do with that energy!

Repeat each of the sentences listed below. You may wish to repeat this activity from time to time as you progress with your wellness program. (You may want to put these statements on a file card for easier reference.)

Before you begin, relax your body by taking three deep cleansing breaths. Breathe in through your nose, hold it for a few seconds, then blow out through your mouth.

A. I forgive myself and acknowledge my power (or higher source power) to achieve my wellness goal. Tomorrow is gone. I'll never go forward if I am only looking back.

B. I forgive others (parents, spouses, associates) and accept that I, not they, am in control of my life. I won't waste precious mental energy placing blame or responsibility outside myself.

C. I am in control of my life. My life is in balance.

CHOICES: TAKING CONTROL OF YOUR LIFE

It is important to understand from the start as you work with this program that everything you do related to your wellness and weight loss should be a matter of choice. If you only do what someone else tells you because you feel you must, not because you want to, you begin to feel manipulated and powerless to control your own life. Frequently the reason weight-loss programs are unsuccessful for an individual is because it becomes impossible for them to not "cheat" based upon a rigid eating regimen they feel they must follow. When you encounter situations where you feel that you have blown it by eating the forbidden cookie and that you have now failed (at least in your mind), the next mental step is why not go ahead and eat the whole package. Nothing you do in the BALANCE program is forbidden. It's all a matter of choice. If you choose to go off your program or, for circumstances that seem beyond your control, you have to or want to eat something you know you shouldn't, it's your own decision.

You are the one in control of your life, not someone else, so you can also choose to make amends and decide to carry on with better choices in the future. When we feel compelled rather than choosing to do something, it can set up a sort of panic feeling or feelings of rebellion. One of the reasons you won't find the word "diet" in this program is because the very use of the word sets up a sort of panic situation with many (myself included) and they tend to start actually craving more to eat than before.

You're not on a diet now. You're involved in making personal choices where nothing is forbidden. Armed with knowledge and techniques, you are able to make choices that work for you rather than against you. You are the one in control, and just knowing this can mean the difference between your perception of success and failure. When you are faced with an eating decision and all you can relate to is "I can't eat this" you experience feelings of deprivation. When you face the same situation from a perspective of "I'm in charge; it's my choice, and instead of the cookie I am going to choose an apple" (for example), you do two things. First, you reinforce the feeling of being in control and thus don't experience the negative aspects associated with failure because you did something that was forbidden. You also create very positive feelings because you are able to make wise choices that help you accomplish what you are trying to achieve. Second, you help your body become accustomed to feeling that it can be as satisfied from eating an apple as it can from eating the cookie. The body and the mind are both learning new tricks and both derive benefit from the decision. It isn't easy, especially at first, but as you begin to achieve more and more success with your choices, it will become easier to make ones that provide you with positive feedback. If you are persuaded to meet every food temptation with the thought "I am forever forbidden," you are much more likely to binge. You will have greater success if you learn to choose or reject food (or amounts of food) knowing the action was your choice and made under circumstances which you controlled such as when you eat whatever, or how much of it you eat. Obviously no matter what gimmick a "diet" seems to promise, you must take in less than you expend. But there are times when the best lesson you can learn is the one you teach yourself; that when you make unwise choices, you don't accomplish your weight loss goals, and what is even more important, you don't feel good about yourself. Feelings of achievement are as important to your overall wellness as losing weight. Rather than viewing your eating and exercise plans as strict inflexible discipline, view them as tools you are using to make changes you want in your life and to accomplish goals you really believe you can achieve. Most of the time it will be your mind rather than your body that's craving something you'd be better off not eating. When you come upon these situations, don't feel you are having to give up something you really want, decide that you would rather choose something that is good for you rather than something that is not.

We have all become conditioned to using food as a reward, as a soother, etc. You have the power to change that conditioning. You can break the connection, the chain, that's tying you to food by learning to do something else rather than eating to soothe anxieties or to promote feelings of well-being. With a little effort, you can learn to use discretion and trade-offs to stay in control. Feeling good about yourself goes hand in hand with feeling in control of your life.

SUPPORT GROUP

There is strong evidence to suggest that a person on a weight-loss program has a greater chance of success if he is actively involved with the support of a peer group. The group plays an important role for its individual members by providing a positive and supportive setting where participants can share experiences and help each other.

Regular contact with a support group can:

• Reinforce motivation and commitment
• Provide a forum for sharing problems and solutions
• Be a source of emotional comfort and encouragement
• Make you aware that others share similar feelings and experiences.

If you do not already have access to a support group, we suggest you start one which can be structured around the topics and information presented in this workbook. While each group will differ because of the wants, needs, and personality of the participants, the following outline provides a framework around which the group can be based.

1. Schedule meetings weekly (or twice a week if that would work better), at a mutually convenient time and location. This could be a public meeting room, a private office, or a home. Some groups function well with lunch meetings, others prefer an evening schedule. An hour to an hour-and-a-half is sufficient.

2. Each member needs to have his own workbook.

3. Meetings can include an individual weight-loss report with each person stating his weight loss (or gain) progress for the week (month). This should be an optional choice for each member of the group. Some groups find a "weigh-in" provides a good motivator.

4. The program should revolve around a different topic each session using a moderator or topic master to provide structure. This person who provides the facilitator role can be changed weekly or be the same person each time. A revolving schedule for this function also works well.

5. The topic for the session can be chosen from those offered in the workbook. Using a periodic guest speaker also works well. After an introduction of the topic by the moderator, each participant should be encouraged to relate his personal experiences and feelings as they relate to the topic. Other group members may choose to offer helpful suggestions or support to each participant's comments.

Although participants should be encouraged to share their feelings, if some individuals choose not to speak (at least at first), the choice should be respected. These groups obviously work best when the members feel comfortable rather than intimidated with the proceedings. While the accommodation process may be slower for some than for others, each member should be encouraged to participate in order to receive the most benefit from the group. Stating their name and their weight-loss objective is at least a beginning. (For instance, "My name is John Doe, my weight-loss goal is 50 pounds. I've been on the program for a month and I've lost 15 pounds.")

6. In addition to the topic chosen for discussion each session, each participant may also choose to relate any special problems he has encountered. The program can be closed with a voice-guided or individual focused relaxation technique where each individual can envision himself as fit and trim. As he relaxes, he should suggest to himself (or the moderator should suggest) that all negative feelings are leaving his body and that he is now enjoying a state of good health and well-being.

The group should attempt to provide an informal, positive and confidential forum where participants can offer and receive support and advice related to their weight-loss experiences. The atmosphere should be one of caring encouragement where no one is required to be an expert, and where participants feel comfortable sharing their feelings.

A WELLNESS PARTNER

Because a support system is an important aspect in helping you achieve your wellness goals, you will want to choose a wellness partner. This person will be in addition to your support group although it could be someone who is also a member of the group. He should be someone (with his approval, of course) you can call or see on a regular basis especially when you feel you are experiencing a crisis or whenever you feel you need some special encouragement.

You might choose to have a joint wellness partner relationship where you each serve as a partner for the other, or you may want to have just a one-way process where you are the one seeking support and advice. You will need to establish guidelines for the relationship between the two of you.

Your wellness partner need not be a specialist or a professional counselor, just another individual who has your best interests at heart and who will offer the quality of advice and support you need. It should, however, be someone with whom you can feel comfortable and whose opinion is one you respect (even though there may be times that you disagree). Above all, it needs to be a relationship based on trust and confidentiality.

As an example, you might establish guidelines where you call your wellness partner daily to review your progress or to preview your wellness plan for the following day (or week). Other instances that will be important are when you are tempted to binge, when you need some special positive reinforcement, and when you need advice or someone with whom to share a concern.

DEVELOP THE BELIEF THAT YOU CAN AND WILL ACHIEVE YOUR GOAL

The underlying concepts involved in achieving a lifestyle change or a wellness/weight-loss goal are basically no different than those you have used before in achieving other goals.

First you must believe that you can achieve the goal. This is not as obvious as it seems. It may become necessary for you to explore your belief or attitudes as they apply to you in relationship with others. If you "say" you want to lose weight, but deep within you feel you are not worthy of being fit and trim, or if you believe that excess weight makes you appear to be strong or powerful, then you will have a conflict. The term "he carries a lot of weight" is a loaded expression if you believe it means that body weight and personal power go hand in hand. In a case where you wish one thing, but deep down believe another, your deeply held beliefs will almost always win.

What may seem to be unconscious thoughts are, in most cases, thoughts that are available to the conscious mind if only you are willing to explore them, accept them, and...where they are aren't working for you...change them. There aren't value or belief systems that are "good" or "bad." There are only those that work well for you and allow you to fulfill your potential or those that keep you from experiencing fulfillment. Denying undesirable behavior doesn't change it. Accepting it and allowing yourself to change and replace the behavior is what will ultimately bring you success.

Each of our thoughts has a result. The same thought repeated over and over will usually have a permanent effect, whether the thought is a positive or a negative one. If you are happy with the effect, then you will seldom examine the thought. Keep in mind that the underlying attitudes that cause our thoughts are not always obvious.

If you find yourself in an experience that is not working for you, then you begin to wonder what's wrong. Why aren't things working for you? It becomes easy to blame others or your background or your job or outside forces, and you begin to accept your negative situation as inevitable because someone else is at fault. It is important for you to acknowledge that you, and no one else, is responsible for what is "you." This doesn't mean that others in the past or present haven't had an impact on you. What it does mean is that if you don't like what you see (or feel), you have the ability to change it. No one else can do it for you. The same ability and power, (whether you believe it is from within you or from a spiritual source) that has allowed you to achieve other successes in your life can also allow you to achieve a weight loss or wellness goal.

Thoughts or beliefs that might seem to be buried in your unconscious mind are available to you. These old responses that aren't working for you can be changed!

It is a matter of choosing to open doors that may appear to be closed and then to examine these thoughts to see if they are responsible for the condition you wish to change. You may need to alter the kinds of messages you are sending yourself, your friends, your family, and your associates. Only by examining your ideas can you learn what you really feel about yourself and find out which ideas have brought you dissatisfaction in your life and which have brought you the results you are pleased with. Use these positive feelings and experiences to reinforce the changes you now wish to make. We perhaps learn best from our mistakes. Instead of regretting them, you can use them as lessons that will help you create new attitudes and new opportunities.

IS THERE A PAYOFF
FOR BEING OVERWEIGHT?

1. These are the payoffs I get for having my weight be an obstacle to relationships.

2. These are all the ways I use overweight to keep from being completely successful.

3. If I woke up tomorrow morning weighing exactly what I wanted to weigh, what three things would I do that I'm not doing now?

4. These are the reasons I like myself exactly the way I am.

II

HEALTH AND NUTRITION

THE WELLNESS CONCEPT

Wellness is a natural state of the body. Unwellness is not. The body naturally seeks a state of wellness as evidenced, for one, by the fact that our systems react to viruses or bacteria without our consciously telling them. When you cut your finger, your body knows how to close and heal the wound. In other words, our bodies have a conscious drive of their own toward wellness that does these things for us. Many diseases are now beginning to be recognized by medical science as conditions where the physical dysfunction is a result of mental processes. This doesn't imply that we are imagining them or thinking them up. What this does tell us is that mental distress can contribute to physical problems such as heart disease, high blood pressure, certain allergic reactions, and lowered immunity to disease. If you are constantly programming negative messages into your system, there is going to be a definite correlation between this and unwellness.

Obesity is one form of unwellness. Men who are 30% overweight have a 70% higher chance of developing coronary heart disease than those at their recommended weight. Men who are 20% overweight are more than twice as likely to develop diabetes, and only a third as likely as a person of normal weight to live to age 80. Other conditions that have been linked to obesity include digestive problems, stroke, respiratory and circulation problems, as well as cancer. The natural state of the body is wellness, as we have said. In its ideal state, the body is not obese. So what are we doing with our minds and our thoughts and our feelings that is causing this unnatural state? This is something that each of you is going to have to discover for himself. There is a direct correlation, however, and this is why we have incorporated into this program a section on behavior/response modification.

If you can begin to modify some of the mental processes that are giving you problems, it's going to have a direct impact on the wellness of your body, because your body is seeking wellness — its natural state. It is necessary to begin focusing on tuning out and changing some of these negative things you're doing to your body. For example, the belief that you have no choice about being overweight is negative thinking. If somewhere along the line you can start to modify that belief system, you're going to have a better chance of success with your wellness program and with weight loss. You must believe that you don't have to be overweight, and then start working on eliminating or modifying some of the other beliefs that no longer work for you. Obesity can be controlled.

We have provided activities and information throughout this workbook to help you identify thoughts and feelings related to the reactions and behaviors you would like to change or modify. We've also given suggestions that will help you accomplish the changes.

WELLNESS GOALS ACTIVITY

1. In my opinion, what does wellness mean as it relates to me?

2. What are my wellness goals?

3. How can the BALANCE program help me achieve these goals?

Continue on the following page with the GETTING TO KNOW ME BETTER activity.

GETTING TO KNOW ME BETTER ACTIVITY

Now examine your belief system as it relates to your wellness goals.

A. What are some of my past successes (with family, friends, career, finances, overcoming obstacles, etc.)

B. What are some strengths that have helped me in the past?

C. What traits or behaviors would I like to change?

D. What do I like most about myself?

E. What do I like least about myself?

F. What are my deepest fears? (i.e., job loss; loss of love of family, friends; loss of health, etc.)

G. Do any of these fears affect my wellness? (List)

H. Do any of these fears affect my weight? (List)

I. If I were not overweight, what in my life would I do differently? (Related to lifestyle, family, job, etc.)

J. I use my excess weight (and/or overeating) as a crutch to keep me from:

K. If I weighed what I believe to be exactly right for my age and my body type, would it make a difference in my life? How?

L. In the past, I believed I couldn't lose weight and keep it off because:

M. I now know I can achieve my weight loss goal because:

WHAT'S A REASONABLE WEIGHT GOAL?

A necessary part of the BALANCE program is making a decision about how much weight you need to lose. This decision should be one that is reasonable and achievable. Your primary focus should be on the state of your physical and mental well-being: how is your excess weight affecting your health at present, and how can losing weight improve the quality of your future health.

While ideal weight charts (see next page) provide some guidelines, you must also take the variables of your specific circumstances into account. Be aware, however, that the excess weight that you may believe makes you look husky and powerful may instead pose a potential threat to your health, especially as you reach your middle years and are less physically active than you were in your youth. Age, however, is no excuse for being unfit. Even individuals who have never exercised regularly can become physically fit and become almost equal to those who have exercised regularly for ten years.

Excess weight can increase your chances of stroke, heart attack and other diseases. At the other end of the spectrum, though, if you have always been very obese, especially for a long period of time, you may never be able to have a 32-inch waist. While excess weight may threaten health, setting unreachable goals can thwart the self esteem which is also necessary for your well-being. A reasonable weight that you can maintain is, in the long run, healthier than a constant "yo-yo" battle where you starve yourself then immediately regain the pounds.

If you have a lot of weight to lose, you may wish to set incremental short-terms goals rather than a seemingly unattainable long-term one. Because of each individual's unique personality, background and physical characteristics, each of you will need to decide for himself what works best.

Learning to like and accept yourself—no matter what you weigh—is important. Seek a balanced goal that will work for you.

DESIRABLE WEIGHT LEVELS FOR MEN

There are several things you need to take into account when you are making a decision about how much you should weigh.

1. Your doctor's opinion (and there is a lot of variance between opinions from doctor to doctor).

2. The size of your frame. A good indicator of this is your wrist size. Many men who are overweight would like to think they have a large frame—they're husky, not fat. However, this is not necessarily the case. Take your wrist measurement to determine your frame size. A small frame has a wrist measurement of from 6-1/2 to 7"; a medium frame from 7 to 7-1/2"; and a large frame from 7-1/2 to 8".

3. You also need to consider the distribution of your excess weight. New biochemical research suggests that the way your weight is distributed over your body is a primary indicator of your cardiovascular health (along with cholesterol levels and blood pressure). If your waist is larger than your hips, you are storing weight within your body cavity. Most women, for instance, tend to put a larger portion of their weight around hips and thighs, and this weight is stored mostly under the skin rather than within the body. Men, however, tend to experience just the opposite. That's why an overweight man's health is at greater risk than a woman with the same percentage of excess weight. I am speaking in general here, of course, but the principle is one that is considered valid. Fat stored within the body acts differently than fat stored under the skin and presents a real health hazard. So, as far as your health is concerned, how your excess weight is distributed over your body may be a better indicator than a weight table.

4. Age is another factor that you should consider. Even though many sources suggest that what you weigh throughout your life should not exceed what was a desirable level for you at age 25, other research suggests that nature may intend for us to have a small gain as we age (as much as 10 pounds every decade, for instance).

The important thing for you to consider is a balanced approach. If you have been extremely overweight for a long time, it may not be reasonable to expect that you will become as trim as you would like. Our bodies, for some perverse reason, seem to hold onto "old" fat harder than "new" fat. Even if you are able to finally attain what you believe is your ideal weight, your body may put up a real battle to maintain that weight. Allowing yourself to stabilize at 10 pounds over your desired weight may be a level you can maintain without having to become a slave to the weight-loss process. Be able to enjoy food AND good health (mental and physical). Achieve BALANCE.

Weight tables/charts, such as the one below, should be used as a guideline only. Other sources who provide weight tables add as much as 10 pounds onto each suggested number.

The table below shows ideal weight ranges for men based on statistics from Metropolitan Life Insurance Co. Weight given is with indoor clothing and shoes with one-inch heels.

HEIGHT	SMALL FRAME	MEDIUM FRAME	LARGE FRAME
5' 2"	128-134	131-141	138-150
5' 3"	130-136	133-143	140-153
5' 4"	132-138	135-145	142-158
5' 5"	134-140	137-148	144-160
5' 6"	136-142	139-151	146-164
5' 7"	138-145	142-154	149-168
5' 8"	140-148	145-157	152-172
5' 9"	142-151	148-160	155-176
5' 10"	144-154	151-163	158-160
5' 11"	146-157	154-166	161-I84
6' 0"	149-160	157-170	164-188
6' 1"	152-164	160-174	168-192
6' 2"	155-168	164-178	172-197
6' 3"	158-172	167-182	176-202
6' 4"	162-176	171-187	181-207

MY WELLNESS CONTRACT AND WEIGHT-LOSS GOAL

I,_____, acknowledge that I am a person with a wellness problem. The effect of this problem is that I overeat and/or eat the wrong foods. This has created a state of unwellness in my body called overweight

I desire and deserve wellness. Therefore, I, _____, make a commitment to myself to use the BALANCE program to help create wellness in my body. As part of this commitment, I choose to eat only those amounts and those kinds of food that will allow me to achieve a weight-loss goal of._____pounds.

I_____, believe in and acknowledge my right to choose wellness and balance in my life.

_____

Signed

_____

Dated

_____

Witnessed (Wellness Partner)

PRELIMINARY EATING ACTIVITY

For one week, keep a record of everything you eat including meals and snacks. (Make extra copies of the log sheet as needed.) In addition to what you will actually eat, you also will need to record when you eat, where you eat, and your mood or emotional state just before eating (i.e., anger, boredom, fright, anxiety, ate out of habit, etc.). Don't plan to be on a weight-loss regimen during this week. What you are trying to do is identify those emotions or places or activities that are triggers for overeating or for eating the wrong foods. Be honest; no one but you will see these sheets.

After you have completed your work sheets (one per day), review them to see if you can determine any specific triggers (i.e., watching TV, being over anxious, tired, tense, etc.).

Look also for food patterns. What kinds of food are you over indulging in: fats, sugar? Is your problem mainly one of quality or quantity—or both?

Try to distinguish if, when you overeat, you were really hungry or if you were feeding your mood. An honest appraisal of your diary can be a valuable tool in planning the next step in the BALANCE program, which is your actual food plan.

At the end of the week, complete the following Preliminary Eating Activity Summary Sheet.

PRELIMINARY EATING ACTIVITY LOG SHEET

WHAT I ATE	WHEN	WHERE	MY MOOD

PRELIMINARY EATING ACTIVITY LOG SHEET

WHAT I ATE	WHEN	WHERE	MY MOOD

PRELIMINARY EATING ACTIVITY LOG SHEET

WHAT I ATE	WHEN	WHERE	MY MOOD

PRELIMINARY EATING ACTIVITY LOG SHEET

WHAT I ATE	WHEN	WHERE	MY MOOD

PRELIMINARY EATING ACTIVITY LOG SHEET

WHAT I ATE	WHEN	WHERE	MY MOOD

PRELIMINARY EATING ACTIVITY LOG SHEET

WHAT I ATE	WHEN	WHERE	MY MOOD

PRELIMINARY EATING ACTIVITY LOG SHEET

WHAT I ATE	WHEN	WHERE	MY MOOD

PRELIMINARY EATING ACTIVITY SUMMARY SHEET

AFTER YOU HAVE KEPT TRACK OF WHAT YOU HAVE BEEN EATING FOR A WEEK, SUMMARIZE YOUR RESULTS.

1. These are the foods I am most likely to overeat that contribute to my overweight situation:

2. I seem to overeat when I am (identify mood or situation):

3. These are foods I've been eating that will sabotage my weight-loss goals:

4. These are foods I could eat instead of those I've listed in #3 above:

5. For me, food seems to be a substitute for:

6. Instead of eating at these times, I could:

HUNGER/FULLNESS ACTIVITY

One problem that may contribute to your overweight is the inability (or loss of ability) to properly respond to hunger cues. Many overeaters seem to have lost the ability to depend upon their internal "appetite monitor" to let them know when they are truly hungry and need food for nourishment or when they are instead seeking food for other reasons. There can also be a problem with your "fullness monitor" so you may not be able to determine the difference between knowing when your body is physically satisfied and when you are continuing to eat to achieve mental satisfaction. This activity may help you by focusing attention on these areas.

Use the scale below to monitor your response to all your meals for a few days. Circle the appropriate number on the scales before and after each meal, and then when you have completed the activity (which should be anywhere from three days to a week), go back and review the results. You will probably want to photocopy extra worksheets. This activity should help you begin to be more aware of your internal mechanisms. Watch to see if you eat meals or snacks when you are not truly hungry, and monitor how you feel when you stop eating. Try to begin to adjust in the future so you don't eat when you don't feel hungry, and so you stop before you are glutted.

BREAKFAST
(before I ate, I felt)

no hunger			**moderate hunger**			**extreme hunger**			
1	2	3	4	5	6	7	8	9	10

(after I stopped eating, I felt)

still hungry			**moderately full**			**glutted**			
1	2	3	4	5	6	7	8	9	10

LUNCH
(before I ate, I felt)

no hunger			**moderate hunger**			**extreme hunger**			
1	2	3	4	5	6	7	8	9	10

(after I stopped eating, I felt)

still hungry			**moderately full**			**glutted**			
1	2	3	4	5	6	7	8	9	10

DINNER
(before I ate, I felt)

no hunger			**moderate hunger**			**extreme hunger**			
1	2	3	4	5	6	7	8	9	10

(after I stopped eating, I felt)

still hungry			**moderately full**			**glutted**			
1	2	3	4	5	6	7	8	9	10

You may also want to monitor any snacks you have during the day in this same manner.

FOOD ADDICTION

There are some interesting correlations between using alcohol, drugs and food as a means of trying to "fix" the problems we encounter. Individuals who have a past history of alcohol or drug abuse, when recovering from these habits, will often replace them with food abuse. Others may have developed a food addiction instead of the alcohol or drug addiction, but the causal factors may be very similar. The common result of all three behaviors is that instead of helping "fix" the problem, they only temporarily dull the pain and they add a very real health hazard.

A look at a typical "why" list of all three abuses points out some similar responses.

YOU MAY OVERINDULGE IN FOOD, ALCOHOL OR DRUGS (OR ALL THREE):

To help relieve feelings of sadness

To reduce anxiety

As a reward

To help you relax

To compensate for sexual problems or frustrations

To reduce fears or inhibitions

As a result of loneliness

As an escape from problems at home or at work

To help you feel more powerful or important

To reduce feelings of inadequacy

There are, however, some better ways of handling these feelings and situations. Simplistically stated, TRY DOING SOMETHING ELSE INSTEAD OF USING FOOD, DRUGS OR ALCOHOL TO SOLVE YOUR PROBLEMS! That, you say, seems obvious. But what, specifically, can you do?

INSTEAD OF OVEREATING, FIND A BETTER WAY TO COPE!

- Communicate your feelings to a non-judgmental listener (i.e., wellness partner, a spouse, a minister, priest or rabbi, a friend, or a professional counselor).

- Exercise. Take a walk. Read a book. Go dancing.

- Do a focused relaxation technique (which can also include tuning into your version of God or a higher power).

- Develop a new hobby, or resurrect an old one. Take a class.

- Take time to smell the flowers. Get outside and enjoy the healing powers of nature.

- Use the "processing" technique. (See *Positive Power of the Mind* section.)

EMOTIONAL OVEREATING ACTIVITY

What you will be trying to learn or define with this activity is whether you are eating from real hunger (actual body hunger) or instead from psychological hunger (to calm anxiety, tensions, sadness, as procrastination, etc.). Once you learn to tell the difference, and once you begin to recognize emotions that cause you to overeat, then you can begin to substitute activities, mental or physical, for the psychological overeating.

Fill out one of the following worksheets (Is Food What I Really Want?) each day for one week when you begin the BALANCE program. You will need to make extra copies of the worksheet. Each time you eat a meal or snack, answer the appropriate questions.

This activity works best as a follow-up to the preliminary eating activity on page 32. In other words, you will spend week one of the BALANCE program filling out that log sheet, and week two filling out the emotional overeating activity sheet. If it seems time consuming and you're anxious to get on with the food plan, consider this. Your excess weight is most likely a condition you have had for some time. You're not going to change your eating and thinking patterns overnight. It is important when driving to a specific destination to first decide your route; consider these week-long "logs" your map to a trim, healthy body. You need to find out just where you are before you can know where you going. Weight loss is not a place -it is a journey, a process. If you skip important steps, you are more likely to sabotage your program than if you progress with a plan. These activities are important components of that plan.

At the end of a week, go back and review each day. Did any one particular emotion seem to show up frequently? If you are encountering stress situations related to your eating patterns, specify what kinds of stress (anger, boredom, anxiety, disappointment, tired, overworked, etc.) Try to identify the emotion(s) that cause you to overeat. If there seem to be too many, focus on only one or two to begin with.

During the week *following* your completion of the worksheets, as you experience that emotion or mood or activity that has in the past caused you to overeat, think about what technique or activity you could substitute for the food. For the next week or two, try to really concentrate on eating only when you are physically hungry and to stop eating when you are physically full. It may take several days before you recognize the difference between "real" hunger and psychological hunger.

Don't worry about what you're going to eat during this period; concentrate only on responding to real hunger (no matter what time of the day it is). Eat *only* when you are truly hungry and substitute an activity for those other times when you would like to eat, but you know you are not genuinely hungry. Activities could include any form of relaxation, exercise, a hobby, etc.

IS FOOD WHAT I REALLY WANT?

DAY # _____

1. Why did I eat this meal?
   Breakfast
   Lunch
   Dinner
   Snacks

2. How did I decide what size portion to eat?

3. How did I decide when I was full or satisfied (what cues did I experience) ?
   Breakfast
   Lunch
   Dinner
   Snacks

4. Before I ate, was I physically hungry or was I psychologically hungry?
   Breakfast
   Lunch
   Dinner
   Snacks

5. How do I recognize my physical hunger, that is, what are the "symptoms" I am interpreting as a hunger signal?
   Breakfast
   Lunch
   Dinner
   Snacks

6. Was I physically full before I finished eating all of my meal (or snack(s)?
   Breakfast
   Lunch
   Dinner
   Snacks

7. Am I substituting food for something else? That is, is there something else I actually want or should do rather than the food (reward myself, calm myself, etc.)?
   Breakfast
   Lunch
   Dinner
   Snacks

8. What time of day did I snack? (Include all snacks during day and evening.)

9. For me, what is the difference between physical hunger and psychological hunger?

10. How does eating from psychological hunger make me feel better?

11. How does eating from psychological hunger make me feel worse?

12. During this day, did I eat something other than what I really wanted to eat?
    Breakfast
    Lunch
    Dinner
    Snacks

MY COMMENTS:

IS FOOD WHAT I REALLY WANT?

DAY # _____

1. Why did I eat this meal?
   Breakfast
   Lunch
   Dinner
   Snacks

2. How did I decide what size portion to eat?

3. How did I decide when I was full or satisfied (what cues did I experience)?
   Breakfast
   Lunch
   Dinner
   Snacks

4. Before I ate, was I physically hungry or was I psychologically hungry?
   Breakfast
   Lunch
   Dinner
   Snacks

5. How do I recognize my physical hunger, that is, what are the "symptoms" I am interpreting as a hunger signal?
   Breakfast
   Lunch
   Dinner
   Snacks

6. Was I physically full before I finished eating all of my meal (or snack(s)?
   Breakfast
   Lunch
   Dinner
   Snacks

7. Am I substituting food for something else? That is, is there something else I actually want or should do rather than the food (reward myself, calm myself, etc.)?
   Breakfast
   Lunch
   Dinner
   Snacks

8. What time of day did I snack? (Include all snacks during day and evening.)

9. For me, what is the difference between physical hunger and psychological hunger?

10. How does eating from psychological hunger make me feel better?

11. How does eating from psychological hunger make me feel worse?

12. During this day, did I eat something other than what I really wanted to eat?
    Breakfast
    Lunch
    Dinner
    Snacks

MY COMMENTS:

IS FOOD WHAT I REALLY WANT?

DAY # _____

1. Why did I eat this meal?
   Breakfast
   Lunch
   Dinner
   Snacks

2. How did I decide what size portion to eat?

3. How did I decide when I was full or satisfied (what cues did I experience)?
   Breakfast
   Lunch
   Dinner
   Snacks

4. Before I ate, was I physically hungry or was I psychologically hungry?
   Breakfast
   Lunch
   Dinner
   Snacks

5. How do I recognize my physical hunger, that is, what are the "symptoms" I am interpreting as a hunger signal?
   Breakfast
   Lunch
   Dinner
   Snacks

6. Was I physically full before I finished eating all of my meal (or snack(s)?
   Breakfast
   Lunch
   Dinner
   Snacks

7. Am I substituting food for something else? That is, is there something else I actually want or should do rather than the food (reward myself, calm myself, etc.)?
   Breakfast
   Lunch
   Dinner
   Snacks

8. What time of day did I snack? (Include all snacks during day and evening.)

9. For me, what is the difference between physical hunger and psychological hunger?

10. How does eating from psychological hunger make me feel better?

11. How does eating from psychological hunger make me feel worse?

12. During this day, did I eat something other than what I really wanted to eat?
    Breakfast
    Lunch
    Dinner
    Snacks

MY COMMENTS:

IS FOOD WHAT I REALLY WANT?

DAY # _____

1. Why did I eat this meal?
    Breakfast
    Lunch
    Dinner
    Snacks

2. How did I decide what size portion to eat?

3. How did I decide when I was full or satisfied (what cues did I experience) ?
    Breakfast
    Lunch
    Dinner
    Snacks

4. Before I ate, was I physically hungry or was I psychologically hungry?
    Breakfast
    Lunch
    Dinner
    Snacks

5. How do I recognize my physical hunger, that is, what are the "symptoms" I am interpreting as a hunger signal?
    Breakfast
    Lunch
    Dinner
    Snacks

6. Was I physically full before I finished eating all of my meal (or snack(s)?
    Breakfast
    Lunch
    Dinner
    Snacks

7. Am I substituting food for something else? That is, is there something else I actually want or should do rather than the food (reward myself, calm myself, etc.)?
    Breakfast
    Lunch
    Dinner
    Snacks

8. What time of day did I snack? (Include all snacks during day and evening.)

9. For me, what is the difference between physical hunger and psychological hunger?

10. How does eating from psychological hunger make me feel better?

11. How does eating from psychological hunger make me feel worse?

12. During this day, did I eat something other than what I really wanted to eat?
    Breakfast
    Lunch
    Dinner
    Snacks

MY COMMENTS:

IS FOOD WHAT I REALLY WANT?

DAY # _____

1. Why did I eat this meal?
   Breakfast
   Lunch
   Dinner
   Snacks

2. How did I decide what size portion to eat?

3. How did I decide when I was full or satisfied (what cues did I experience) ?
   Breakfast
   Lunch
   Dinner
   Snacks

4. Before I ate, was I physically hungry or was I psychologically hungry?
   Breakfast
   Lunch
   Dinner
   Snacks

5. How do I recognize my physical hunger, that is, what are the "symptoms" I am interpreting as a hunger signal?
   Breakfast
   Lunch
   Dinner
   Snacks

6. Was I physically full before I finished eating all of my meal (or snack(s)?
   Breakfast
   Lunch
   Dinner
   Snacks

7. Am I substituting food for something else? That is, is there something else I actually want or should do rather than the food (reward myself, calm myself, etc.)?
   Breakfast
   Lunch
   Dinner
   Snacks

8. What time of day did I snack? (Include all snacks during day and evening.)

9. For me, what is the difference between physical hunger and psychological hunger?

10. How does eating from psychological hunger make me feel better?

11. How does eating from psychological hunger make me feel worse?

12. During this day, did I eat something other than what I really wanted to eat?
    Breakfast
    Lunch
    Dinner
    Snacks

MY COMMENTS:

IS FOOD WHAT I REALLY WANT?

DAY # _____

1. Why did I eat this meal?
    Breakfast
    Lunch
    Dinner
    Snacks

2. How did I decide what size portion to eat?

3. How did I decide when I was full or satisfied (what cues did I experience)?
    Breakfast
    Lunch
    Dinner
    Snacks

4. Before I ate, was I physically hungry or was I psychologically hungry?
    Breakfast
    Lunch
    Dinner
    Snacks

5. How do I recognize my physical hunger, that is, what are the "symptoms" I am interpreting as a hunger signal?
    Breakfast
    Lunch
    Dinner
    Snacks

6. Was I physically full before I finished eating all of my meal (or snack(s)?
    Breakfast
    Lunch
    Dinner
    Snacks

7. Am I substituting food for something else? That is, is there something else I actually want or should do rather than the food (reward myself, calm myself, etc.)?
    Breakfast
    Lunch
    Dinner
    Snacks

8. What time of day did I snack? (Include all snacks during day and evening.)

9. For me, what is the difference between physical hunger and psychological hunger?

10. How does eating from psychological hunger make me feel better?

11. How does eating from psychological hunger make me feel worse?

12. During this day, did I eat something other than what I really wanted to eat?
    Breakfast
    Lunch
    Dinner
    Snacks

MY COMMENTS:

IS FOOD WHAT I REALLY WANT?

DAY # _____

1. Why did I eat this meal?
   Breakfast
   Lunch
   Dinner
   Snacks

2. How did I decide what size portion to eat?

3. How did I decide when I was full or satisfied (what cues did I experience) ?
   Breakfast
   Lunch
   Dinner
   Snacks

4. Before I ate, was I physically hungry or was I psychologically hungry?
   Breakfast
   Lunch
   Dinner
   Snacks

5. How do I recognize my physical hunger, that is, what are the "symptoms" I am interpreting as a hunger signal?
   Breakfast
   Lunch
   Dinner
   Snacks

6. Was I physically full before I finished eating all of my meal (or snack(s)?
   Breakfast
   Lunch
   Dinner
   Snacks

7. Am I substituting food for something else? That is, is there something else I actually want or should do rather than the food (reward myself, calm myself, etc.)?
   Breakfast
   Lunch
   Dinner
   Snacks

8. What time of day did I snack? (Include all snacks during day and evening.)

9. For me, what is the difference between physical hunger and psychological hunger?

10. How does eating from psychological hunger make me feel better?

11. How does eating from psychological hunger make me feel worse?

12. During this day, did I eat something other than what I really wanted to eat?
Breakfast
Lunch
Dinner
Snacks

MY COMMENTS:

SET POINT OR BASAL METABOLIC RATE (BMR)

A repeated weight loss/weight gain pattern is called the yo-yo syndrome. This is what is happening when you lose 10 or more pounds, then all too quickly gain back all of it and then some. If you repeat this cycle over and over again, you are actually increasing your body's ability to store and produce more fat! Even a brief crash diet can trigger this response, and the effects can last for months and years.

Why does this happen? Because when you deprive your body of its ideal maintenance calories by crash dieting, it starts to turn down your basal metabolic rate, or set point, which is the rate at which your body burns calories when at rest. The body, on its own—without any conscious input from you—involuntarily reacts to what it perceives to be a "starvation" condition and starts to burn fewer and fewer calories. Your BMR can actually drop by as much as 10 to 50 percent.

Now when you return to eating what should be a normal maintenance intake, your body immediately hoards this new food supply in its fat reserve. It doesn't know it is not still in a state of starvation. It's as if it can't depend upon a regular supply of food, so it has prepared itself to store fat in case it is needed for another "starvation" situation. That's why you yo-yo; that's why you gain weight back so fast after crash dieting even though you aren't overeating.

Each time you put your body through this cycle, you drop your BMR even lower so it can survive on fewer and fewer calories. You will continue to burn fewer calories after dieting than you did before you started dieting. Your body's involuntary survival mechanism has now turned into a fat factory! You will also increase your fat-to-muscle ratio.

The good news is that the process can be reversed. Your set point can be raised and the dieting damage undone. The solution is regular physical activity and a healthy food plan. This is why exercise is so important to your wellness plan. It actually serves a three-fold purpose:

1. It will help you eliminate the yo-yo syndrome by stabilizing (or raising) your BMR.

2. It will help you build or keep muscle tone so that your body will be firmer and more attractive.

3. By building or increasing your muscle mass, you will actually be able to eat more and stay slim. Muscle burns more calories than fat. Therefore, the greater the muscle proportion of your body weight, the more fuel your system will burn and the more you can eat without gaining weight. This is why exercise is crucial for weight loss as well as for maintaining a desirable weight level.

III

FOOD AND EATING

WHAT IS FOOD
FOOD AS A NUTRIENT

In order to help simplify the understanding and use of food from a nutritional aspect, food is categorized into three classifications. What we eat is composed of various proportions or combinations of what are referred to as nutrients. All food contains one or more of the following:

*   FATS

*   CARBOHYDRATES

*   PROTEIN

You need a certain amount of each of these nutrients in order to maintain good health and for your body to operate in a functional, efficient manner. Adult nutritional needs differ from those of growing children. As far as your body is concerned, not all food is created equal. While you might assume a calorie is a calorie (no matter its nutrient content,) your body makes a discrimination. Fat, for instance, has 9 calories per gram whereas protein and carbohydrates each have only 4 calories per gram. Also, eating 800 calories of fat will not be processed by your body in the same way as 800 calories of complex (unrefined) carbohydrates, such as an apple. The fat calories tend to be stored as body fat, while the complex carbohydrates and protein, unless they exceed your nutritional requirements, will be used up as energy. This is an oversimplification, but will suffice for now. The objective is to keep your fat intake low to lose weight and maintain wellness.

In addition to the composition of foods given above, food is also nutritionally classified as food groups, of which there are four. Those include:

• Meat, fish, poultry and dried beans (plus eggs, seeds, nuts) - contain protein and fat content

• Dairy foods (milk, cheese, butter, yogurt) - contain protein and fat

• Fruits and vegetables - unrefined carbohydrates

• Bread and cereal (including rice, pasta, grains) mostly unrefined carbohydrates

Recently, in an effort to focus on our need for less fat as well as the beneficial health aspects of eating more complex carbohydrates, the traditional four food groups are being restructured. Health researchers now advocate a group pyramid as a suggested guideline. The top of the pyramid suggests fats, oil and sweets be used sparingly and that we increase our consumption of fruits, vegetables and grains.

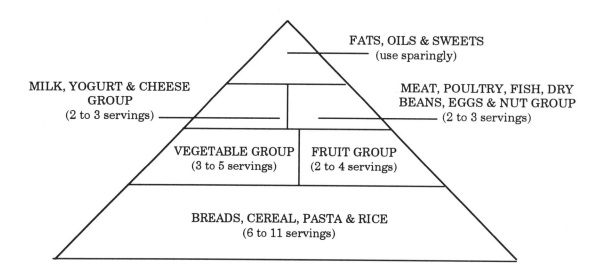

The pyramid format seems to have some deficiencies from my point of view. First, it would be more easily comprehended if the "bad stuff" were at the bottom and the "good stuff" at the top, so I'd like to see an inverted pyramid. Second, milk, yogurt and cheese are lumped together. There's a big difference between "regular" versions of these versus the low-fat and non-fat version. The non-fat version won't attack your arteries. The high-fat kind may. Finally, for anyone trying to lose weight, the number of servings of bread, cereal, rice and pasta may be excessive. Also, they don't make clear how much a "serving" is.

At any rate, it is a suggested guide that tries to focus our attention on the real need for Americans to become more knowledgeable about the close connection between what we eat and the state of our health—something traditional medicine in this country has been slow to recognize.

WHAT IS A CALORIE?

A calorie is a unit of measure to describe the amount of energy it takes to utilize food. The calories measure heat released by energy.

Your body requires a specific amount of calories to function. Simplistically stated, when you take in more than this amount, you gain weight. When you take in less, you lose weight. There are various factors that determine what you, as an individual, can consume in the form of calories in order to maintain a desired weight level. Your age, your level of physical activity, your basal metabolic rate, and your body size all affect how many calories you can consume to either lose, gain, or maintain weight.

One pound of body fat is the equivalent of 3,500 calories. In order to lose a pound, you will need to consume 3,500 fewer calories than are required to maintain your weight. For instance, if you are active, between 35 and 55 years of age, and weigh 187 pounds, you would be able to eat about 3,000 calories per day to maintain that weight. If you wish to lose weight, you would need to drop 3,500 calories to lose one pound. You need to reduce your daily food intake, but you should not eat fewer than 1,400 to 1,600 calories in any one day. Thus, it will take about a week to lose 3 to 4 pounds.

This system is approximate and not an exact measurement, so it will differ somewhat from person to person because your basal metabolisms differ.

Weight loss also includes a certain amount of water loss, which is what you primarily lose early in your weight-loss cycle. Some weeks you will plateau and not seem to lose anything (at least according to your scales). This is a natural phenomenon and should not be viewed as discouraging or as failure. Continue to stick with your plan and you will lose. Also, weight loss patterns shouldn't be expected to go down in a straight diagonal line. It will instead more likely be a zig-zag pattern. There are going to be times, for whatever reason, that you will go off your plan for a short time. This is also normal. When this does occur, don't berate yourself or count this as a failure. Consider it part of your planned zig-zag pattern and get back on the plan, then stick with it. It takes time, but it will work if you want it to.

EXAMPLE:

TO MAINTAIN DESIRED WEIGHT - 187 POUNDS
3,000 calories X 7 days = **21,000** calories a week

YOUR FOOD PLAN
1,500 calories X 7 days = **10,500** calories a week

CALORIE REDUCTION

21,000 calories minus **10,500** calories =

10,500 calories divided by 3,500 calories =

Weight loss of 3 pounds

Remember that this is simply a guide. Your system may deviate from the norm. It is extremely important to weigh and measure what you eat in order to determine your correct caloric intake.

It is also extremely important to become familiar with the kinds of calories you are eating. Calories from protein and unrefined carbohydrates, such as fruit and vegetables, help keep you healthy; too many fat calories will sabotage both health and weight-loss efforts. You need to know which kinds of calories work best for optimum health.

FATS, SUGAR AND SALT

Fats, sugar and salt are three major contributors to "food addictions." These addictions can be tough habits to break because most of us have become accustomed to eating large quantities of each, especially in processed food.

FATS

From both a health and a chemical standpoint, not all fats are alike. They can be defined as belonging to three categories: saturated, polyunsaturated, and monounsaturated. In addition to wanting to limit your intake of fats (which also includes oils) from a weight-loss aspect, there is now mounting evidence that too much of the wrong kind of fat is a prime contributor to high cholesterol levels in the bloodstream. Remember that your body manufactures its own cholesterol from the fat products you eat. So, even if a particular food contains no cholesterol, but has a lot of fat, it is just as bad for you as eating cholesterol. Eating a lot of food that contains high amounts of both cholesterol and saturated fat can be potentially harmful. This means that even when you reach your weight-loss goal, you will want to continue monitoring your intake of fats from a wellness standpoint.

Fat (or oil) is classified into three types. All contain the same amount of calories—100 per tablespoon (9 calories per gram).

Saturated Fats

This kind of fat comes mainly from animal sources (beef, lamb, and pork) as well as from chicken and fish and is also found in eggs, butter, whole milk and cheese. The amount of saturated fat in beef and pork is somewhat less their total fat content. Many stores now carry a "light" variety of beef which has both fewer total calories and fewer saturated fat grams than regular cuts of beef. USDA labeling requires that "light" beef have no more than 10% fat or at least 25% less fat than averages for similar cuts. Coconut, palm, and palm kernel oil (also referred to as tropical oils) are also highly saturated. These oils, because they are inexpensive, abound in commercially prepared foods. This is one of the reasons why it is important for you to try to use fresh food whenever possible, and it is also why you will need to learn to read food labels. Some of the foods to watch out for that contain high amounts of this kind of fat are processed meats (hot dogs, lunch meat, sausage), ice cream, egg yolks, hard cheese, cream, and coffee "creamers". For the sake of your waistline and your health, try to remove as much saturated fat from your food plan as possible—now and forever.

Polyunsaturated Fats

Evidence indicates that this kind of fat, found mostly in oil, is not as dangerous to the arteries. However, it does contain the same amount of calories, so you will want to watch closely how much you consume. Within this category are corn, cottonseed, safflower, soybean and sunflower oils. Fish oil also falls within this category but is somewhat different because it also contains a beneficial fatty acid called omega 3 which scientists now think helps reduce blood cholesterol. Canola oil, soybeans, walnuts and wheat germ are also sources of omega 3.

Monounsaturated Fats

From a health standpoint, these kinds of fats may be the most desirable. They include olive, peanut, and canola oils. Evidence suggests these oils may possibly help lower total cholesterol levels. In a weight-loss program, no more than 10% to 20% of your total calories should be from oil, and that oil should come from the monounsaturated category if possible. One tablespoon daily is as much as your body needs while you are on a weight-loss regimen.

Your best fat choices from a weight-loss standpoint as well as from a health standpoint include fish, buttermilk, non-fat yogurt and skim milk. Also be aware that "cholesterol free" doesn't mean fat free, and products with this term on their packaging many times contain high amounts of saturated fat.

The American Heart Association suggests the following guidelines:

1. Total fat should be less than 30% of calories.

2. Saturated fat should account for less than 10% of calories.

3. Polyunsaturated fat should not exceed 10% of calories.

4. Cholesterol should not exceed 300 milligrams a day.

5. Sodium should not exceed 3,000 milligrams a day.

SUGAR

A great many commercially prepared foods contain sugar in one of its various forms such as sucrose, corn syrup, and dextrose, for example. While the Food and Drug Administration recognizes these sugars as safe, there is some controversy among nutritionists as to just how much is healthy. High in calories (16 calories per level teaspoon), and low on nutrition (especially refined "table" sugar), there doesn't seem to be much benefit. However, because of its taste appeal, most of us have gotten used to eating a lot of it, sometimes unknowingly. For instance, there are approximately 9 teaspoons of sugar in a 12-ounce soft drink. Most breakfast cereals contain high amounts of sugar (this is in addition to what you will add from your sugar bowl). Consequently, it's not surprising that so many of us are addicted to the taste, and that the more we eat the more desensitized our taste buds become; thus, the more we use in our food. Sugar has also been linked to the storage of body fat.

Because alcohol turns to sugar in the blood stream, the addiction to this substance is easily transferred by the recovering alcoholic to a desire for sweets (in any of its forms). Those who have other diseases where sugar causes havoc with the system include diabetics and those with hypoglycemia. There have been studies which suggest that an over abundance of sugar in the diets of some children can cause hyper kinetic activity with its attendant symptoms which can range from lack of ability to concentrate all the way to personality disorders.

While sugar is a quick energy booster, it only temporarily raises the glucose (sugar) level in your blood. Your pancreas then starts pouring out insulin to compensate, and you can end up with extreme swings that adversely affect not only your appetite, but even your personality. The exception to this effect is a natural sugar called fructose, which is found in fruits. This kind of sugar can actually help stabilize appetite swings because is helps stabilize blood sugar levels.

We suggest that no matter which food plan you choose, that you try as much as possible to eliminate, or at least moderate, sugar (except that found naturally in fruit and vegetables) from your food plan. In addition to decreasing your calorie intake, you need to direct your appetite away from a craving for sweets. Most products containing high sugar content also contain high fat content (i.e., baked goods, ice cream, etc.). You can reeducate your palate by trying to eliminate these products and replace them with fresh fruit. Moderate amounts of frozen non-fat yogurt that includes fruit is just as tasty as ice cream and won't sabotage your weight loss and arteries. Whole fruits are preferable to juice as they contain fewer calories and necessary fiber. A glass of orange juice has 100 calories and no fiber, while the whole orange has only 60 calories plus fiber. The fiber helps you feel full as well as providing other significant health benefits.

SALT

You're likely to find as many opinions on salt consumption as you find sources. However, a viewpoint shared by most nutrition and medical experts is that we get more than we need, especially when we are eating a lot of processed food. Salt (sodium) is a preservative, it enhances taste, and it's not expensive, so you will find a lot of it in virtually all processed food. The desire for salty food is an acquired taste, and you can retrain yourself to like less salt. In its natural sodium form, it's everywhere, even in water. While it is estimated that only one in five has health-related problems from sodium-chloride consumption, nonetheless, it in considered to be a contributing factor for many with high blood pressure. About half of those with hypertension find their blood pressure is affected by salt consumption. The USDA guidelines recommend between 1,100 and 3,300 milligrams of sodium per day. You and your doctor should be the ones to make a determination related to your sodium intake.

CHOLESTEROL

Today, most if not all of us have added the word cholesterol to our vocabularies. But what does this word mean as it relates to your situation?

Elevated cholesterol is a significant culprit in the development of coronary heart disease. it can be a killer—a time bomb in your veins! You need to know how your levels can affect your state of wellness. This can only be determined by a blood test. If your total cholesterol level is too high, there are things you can do to lower it...modified eating, exercise and stress reduction. Even if it's not high at the moment, you still may want to undertake some moderate steps to protect yourself in the future.

In very simple terms, cholesterol is a fatty substance produced in your liver and carried in your bloodstream. You produce it from the fat you eat. Cholesterol is also present in animal products (meat, eggs, dairy products). In general, other foods such as fruits and vegetables don't contain cholesterol. So, your cholesterol level is a combination of what you eat plus what your own body produces. When your levels get too high, the excess amounts coat and plug the lining of your blood vessels and can cause devastating health problems.

There are two kinds of cholesterol, one called high density lipoproteins (HDL) and the other called low density lipoproteins (LDL). High HDL levels are considered to be "good" cholesterol, while high LDL levels are cause for concern. The ration between these factors are of prime importance. A blood test is needed to diagnose the ratio of the two types. The excess amounts of LDL cholesterol become deposits (called plaque) that can cause health problems such as athero-sclerosis, which is a hardening or closing of the arteries. Most of us will tend to have some degree of atherosclerosis as part of the aging process, but if kept to a minimum, it won't cause troublesome symptoms. However, the National Institutes of Health has estimated that half of all adult Americans have blood cholesterol levels that could lead to heart disease.

This is why you need to be concerned about the amount of dietary cholesterol you eat. The American Heart Association recommends no more than 300 milligrams per day. Some individuals seem to be more prone than others (through genetically inherited tendencies, for instance) to elevated cholesterol levels. Medical experts consider total levels above 200 to be cause for some concern. Many believe the desired level should be around 180. Levels above 240 are potentially dangerous. These cholesterol levels can be lowered with a modified diet low in dietary cholesterol. We strongly suggest that you consult your physician to determine your present levels. If you do need to be on a restricted diet to lower cholesterol, this can still be incorporated into a weight-loss food plan.

As a preventive measure, we encourage you to follow guidelines established by the American Heart Association (see section on Eating Nutritionally). If you can maintain a level of 150, which is well below the American average of 220, your risk of heart attack is ten times less than average.

Your total cholesterol level, however, is but one factor in determining if you have artery problems related to heart disease. It is also important to take into account how high your HDL level is (for instance for a man between 40 and 59 years of age, an HDL rating of over 52 is considered excellent and less than 37 is considered high risk). If your total cholesterol level is a bit high, but your HDL level is also high, you are at less risk than if your HDL level was low. A ratio between HDL and total cholesterol levels (divide total cholesterol by HDL) of from 2.6 to 4.2 is considered excellent in the 40 to 59-year-old category, while a ratio of 6.1 or higher is cause for some concern.

It's important to know that your body must take in a certain amount of fat in order to function properly. Also, a certain balance of cholesterol is necessary to your body. So, we must eat fat in some form, and we also must produce some cholesterol. As in all other things... BALANCE is the key concept.

THE LABELING GAME

Present food labeling practices allow for a lot of misleading and/or confusing information, or in many cases, lack of information. New labeling laws have been established that will require manufacturers to be much more open and accurate about their products' contents. But until these new requirements bring about actual changes in the labels of the food on your grocery store's shelves (starting mid-1993 and required by May 1994), you need to learn to scrutinize labeling information in order to make wise choices about what you eat.

One recent change you will now see when you are shopping relates to a seal of approval from the American Heart Association. Called a HeartGuide, these red heart-shaped seals are on products that have been tested and that meet criteria based on the AHA's guidelines for fat, cholesterol and sodium. One potential problem with this seal is the fact that the food manufacturers have to apply and pay a significant fee to get this seal placed on their products. There are many smaller food suppliers, those who are local for instance, that simply can't afford to purchase this seal, but whose products meet the standards. Therefore, the implication that displaying the seal makes some products preferable to others can be misleading.

When you are on a weight-loss food plan, it is particularly important to be aware of how much dietary fat you are eating. If you can reduce the amount of fat you eat to 10% of your total daily calories, you will have a much easier and healthier weight loss result. (As stated earlier, nutrition and health experts suggest that even if you are not on a weight-loss regimen that no more than 30% of your calories should come from fat.) Because following these guidelines is so important, you need to become aware of what the percentages given on labels actually mean.

Fat doesn't weigh much, but it is very calorie dense. A half cup of vegetable oil, for instance, weighs less than a half cup of rice; but the oil has about 1,000 calories, while the same amount of cooked rice has only 92 calories. (Fat contains 9 calories per gram.) Also, vegetable oils differ greatly in their saturated fat content. Remember that your body turns saturated fat into cholesterol. Canola oil, which is a monounsaturated oil, contains only 7% saturated fat, while polyunsaturated fats such as corn, olive and soybean oil contain from 13% to 15% saturated fat. Even higher in fat content, stick margarines average 26% while palm oil has 52%, palm kernel oil 86%, and coconut oils a whopping 92% saturated fat. Many food manufacturers probably hope you aren't aware of these percentages. For instance, many of the foods you would think are healthy are actually laced with saturated oils, but you won't be aware of it unless you get adept at label reading, and even then, much of the information isn't given.

Fat percentages given on packages can be misleading. If a food claims to be 80% fat free, that means 80% of the product's total weight is fat free-not 80% of its calories. This can make a big difference when you are doing a meal plan. Two percent milk, for instance, gets 35% of its total calories from fat. (To figure what percentage of fat is in a food product, you will need to know per serving the number of fat grams and the number of calories. Example: There are 120 calories and 4.7 grams of fat in an 8 ounce glass of 2% milk. Multiply the 4.7 fat grams by 9 calories per gram and you get 42.3. These are the fat calories in the glass of milk. Now divide 42.3 by 120, which are the total calories in the glass of milk, and you get 35%.) A food that has over 30% of its calories from fat is considered a high-fat food. Check the fat grams per serving rather than focusing on the fact that the product lays claim to a low percentage of its weight from fat.

One requirement of labeling is that contents much be listed in descending order—from most to least. This means that if sugar is the first ingredient listed, the product contains more sugar than whatever else is in the food. Again, be aware that sugar is only one word used to indicate a sweetening ingredient. (Glucose, fructose, corn syrup, honey. etc. all contain just as many, if not more, calories than sugar. A product can contain one of more of these ingredients and still bear a "sugar-free" label.)

Another booby trap to beware of is "serving size". Various ice cream-type products boldly display a seemingly low calorie per serving label, (80 or 100 calories, for instance) but when you check out the serving size, you'll find it may only be 3 ounces—a pretty small serving indeed. The same with breakfast cereals. Many cereals list 110 calories per serving but when you check out the serving size, you'll find it varies from 1/2 to 1-1/2 cups. If you're going for quantity, opt for the larger volume for the same calories.

Many "low calorie" frozen dinners are similar in calorie count (under 300 calories), but they vary considerably in fat content. Among different brands of these dinners, the percent of calories from fat varies from 13% to 32% (or from 3.8 to 10.8 grams of fat per serving). Multiply fat grams by 9 to convert to calories. If you choose to eat these entrees, select those that have the smallest percentage of fat grams.

A particularly misleading term showing up on packaging is the bold statement "no cholesterol." While they may contain no dietary cholesterol, many of these products contain high amounts of "tropical oil" that your body will convert to cholesterol. At the present time, most food labels don't specify how much of the fat in the product is saturated and how much is unsaturated, so beware!

While improved labeling will allow consumers to more easily tell specifically how much and what type of fat the product contains, you will still want to scrutinize product contents. The labels will still need interpretation based upon the percentage of fat you intend to eat in your daily fare (not over 20% total for the day while on weight loss). The nutrition information given does not take into account that most men need 2500 maintenance calories nor do they give recommendations of what they term "daily values" for children or the elderly. Also many medical authorities believe the suggested 30% fat consumption figure may be too high for preventing heart disease and other illness.

The more proficient you become at analyzing the content of the food you are eating, the better control you will have over what you eat. Eating food in its fresh, natural form (fresh vegetables and fruit, for instance) means you won't be subjected to questionable labeling practices.

WATER, COFFEE AND ALCOHOL

WATER

Almost without exception, all diet plans emphasize drinking from eight to ten glasses of water (or more) per day. Extensive research has been done on the benefits of drinking water in connection with weight loss, and evidence shows that drinking this suggested amount of water accelerates the rate of flushing fat out of your system.

More than half your body is water—around 50 quarts—and losing even a small percentage of this through the hard breathing and perspiration that comes from exercise can have an adverse effect on your body. Drinking water can help curb your appetite and also aids digestion. Adequate water is especially important when you are exercising because it helps cool your body and lubricates your joints. Other health benefits provided by drinking water include flushing out waste products and carrying nutrients to you cells.

We strongly recommend that you incorporate water into your wellness program. For those who are not used to drinking this much water (and especially individuals in office situations), it may be easier for you to remember to pour and drink half a glass or more each hour. This way it doesn't seem like you are having to drink so much or to force so much down at one time. If you have some resistance to tap water, try seltzer or mineral water with a little lemon or lime juice. Also try substituting water for the coffee you normally drink throughout the day.

COFFEE

Various studies indicate that caffeine tends to cause an appetite increase for many individuals. A high level of caffeine in the system also tends to make you more jittery because caffeine is a stimulant. Particularly when you are taking in less food than you are used to, and your natural inclination may be to substitute coffee for food. If you drink too much you are going to severely agitate your nervous system. If you can, try to limit your coffee consumption. A cup of tea has much less caffeine than coffee, but even too much of that may be more stimulant than you need at this time.

We're not suggesting that you totally do away with coffee (or tea), because you're probably going to have enough of a problem doing without your usual quantity of food. To add the additional stress of completely doing away with caffeine (if you're used to a substantial amount), can be extremely uncomfortable for you. However, do try to gradually cut back your caffeine consumption to just one or two cups a day. This will help reduce the normal coffee jitters and in the long run be much healthier for you. Drinking coffee, by the way, does not replace the need to drink water.

If you feel you must add cream and/or sugar, try substituting dry powdered milk (*not* dry "creamer" products containing tropical oils) or skim milk in place of the cream, and use sugar substitute in place of sugar. Go easy on these, however. The calories add up when you drink several cups per day, and these calories shouldn't take the place of the nutrients your body needs.

ALCOHOL

There have been several studies recently related to the correlation between alcohol and weight. What these studies suggest is that, total calorie assumption aside, you **will** have a tendency to gain more weight if you drink than if you do not. The reason is that alcohol affects your body's metabolic rate. In other words, your body becomes less efficient in burning calories from food if you drink alcohol.

Other studies, especially some done in France, are taking a look at the effect of alcohol on our arteries. There seems to be some evidence, albeit controversial, that drinking red wine may have health benefits. Some countries such as France and Japan, where alcohol consumption is fairly high, have much lower death rates from coronary problems. However, other factors such as diet may be part of the equation.

In any event, you must decide what is best for you. The mounting evidence that alcohol affects the weight gain/weight loss process seems sufficient enough to suggest that you do not drink alcohol at all during the period when you are trying to lose weight, and that you drink only in moderation when you are trying to maintain your weight level.

MODERATE FOODS

(CAN BE ADDED DURING MAINTENANCE)

During the weight-loss portion of your wellness program, you will lose weight more efficiently if you avoid certain foods. Remember, however, there are no forbidden foods. Perceiving food from that perspective tends to trigger feelings of deprivation which is not where you should be headed. A better, more productive viewpoint is to realize that you have the power of choice over what you eat and to become aware that some foods work less effectively than others for losing weight. Allow yourself to control food rather than allowing food to control you. These foods can be added in *reasonable quantities* during the maintenance portion of your program. Remember, eating too much and eating foods that contain high amounts of fat and refined carbohydrates (white flour, sugar), are what have contributed to your overweight situation. Try to stick with fresh rather than commercially prepared food whenever possible.

MODERATE FRUIT FOODS

Cherries, figs, dates, grapes, any juices containing added sugar

MODERATE VEGETABLE FOODS

Dry beans (such as lima, kidney, pinto, navy), corn and peas. These are excellent sources of fiber, but higher in calories than other veggies, so need to be eaten with some degree of moderation.

MODERATE GRAIN FOODS

Any packaged cold cereal with added sugar, chips, crackers (except low-fat types such as Wasa bread, Swedish flatbread, etc.)

MODERATE PROTEIN FOODS

Oily or salted fish (i.e., any fish that is canned or packaged in oil. Water packed is okay); packaged lunch meats and wieners; any meat with high fat content such as sausage, bacon, etc.

MODERATE DAIRY FOODS

Cream, ice cream, whole milk, cheese (except a bit of grated Parmesan or Romano for flavoring), coffee creamers

MISCELLANEOUS

Alcohol (on maintenance limit to two drinks per day maximum)

Desserts containing white flour, fats and/or sugar (pie, cake, cookies)

Oils and fats (except for that specifically allowed on your food plan)

Prepared salad dressings containing oil or sugar

Syrup (use sparingly or use a sugar-free variety)

Avocados and olives

Nuts and seeds

Candy, jams and jellies (use sparingly or those with no added sugar)

Sauces containing sugar or fat

THINK WITH YOUR BRAIN, NOT WITH YOUR STOMACH!

SUPER FOODS

In other parts of this book we have presented guidelines about foods to avoid, both from a standpoint of health and to enable you to lose weight. Therefore, you may be encouraged to know there are also foods you should seek out which seem to have special qualities that can help you stay healthy as well as help you lose and keep off pounds. Chief among these are the fiber foods —fruits, vegetables and grain products. In addition to essential vitamins and minerals, these super foods contain either soluble or insoluble fiber, sometimes both. Each type of fiber has health advantages. While many foods have nutritional benefits, there appear to certain ones that are "super" good for you.

FRUIT

All varieties of fruit are good for you, but an apple seems to have almost magical qualities. It, perhaps better than almost any other fruit or vegetable, can stabilize your blood sugar because of its ability to keep blood-glucose levels steadier for a longer time. This means that you are less likely to feel hungry between meals. The pectin in apples also helps clear cholesterol from your bloodstream and helps lower blood pressure. There is also evidence that eating apples regularly can result in fewer upper respiratory infections.

Kiwi fruit, which is only beginning to acquire recognition in this country, it is definitely worth adding to your eating regimen. Kiwi is higher in fiber than bran flakes, has more vitamin C than an orange, and more vitamin E than an avocado while still being low in calories.

Bananas protect the stomach lining from irritation by aspirin and certain other drugs and appear to provide some relief for indigestion problems. For many, bananas have also been successful in treating certain ulcer symptoms.

VEGETABLES

Broccoli, carrots, green pepper, cabbage, cauliflower, in fact all dark green and orange vegetables, have been found to lower many kinds of cancer risk such as colon, pancreas and lung cancer. Green pepper seems to have a connection with lowering cholesterol levels. Carrots are rich in beta carotene, a cancer fighter. Broccoli heads the list of vegetables rich in calcium as well as vitamins A and C. All are low in calories and high in nutrients and should be included in your food plan.

Not only do onions and garlic add taste and variety to your recipes, they have health benefits as well. Onions can boost your HDL (good) cholesterol levels and help lower total cholesterol levels.

They also help regulate blood sugar levels (which stabilizes your appetite). The National Cancer Institute is also finding evidence that both onions and garlic may help prevent certain kinds of cancer.

WHOLE GRAINS AND BRAN

Grandma knew oatmeal was good for you, but probably didn't know exactly why. Now medical science has gotten on the bandwagon. Daily consumption of bran such as that found in oats, wheat, rice, barley, and corn all provide some important health benefits. Food containing these brans (such as hot and cold cereals) may also keep you feeling fuller longer than many other foods, so they make an excellent breakfast choice. A high-fiber breakfast will very likely make you feel less hungry at lunch time. (Beware, however, of cold packaged cereals that contain highly saturated tropical oils such as coconut or palm oil, as well as excessive sugar and sodium.)

Soluble fiber such as that found in oats and barley help lower cholesterol, while insoluble fiber such as that found in rice, corn and wheat help prevent constipation and may also protect against colon cancer. Both soluble and insoluble fiber are important, so be sure to eat a variety that includes each.

You need to be aware that there is a lot of packaging and advertising hype going on regarding dietary fiber, especially oat bran. While oat bran quite probably has health benefits, so do other kinds of brans such as rice, etc. Many products such as bread, frozen waffles, muffins, etc. are stating they contain oat bran, which they do; however the quantity within the products is so small in most cases that you would have to eat a tremendous amount to get the health benefits their labeling implies. Also, these products are likely to be high in fat and sugar content. Compare labels for "per serving" grams when you're considering adding bran to your meals.

FISH

An enzyme found in cold-water fish sources (omega 3) has been linked with lowered susceptibility to heart disease. Omega-3 rich seafood may also help prevent certain kinds of cancer, provide arthritis relief, and help regulate our immune systems. (Fish oil supplements, by the way, have not been proven to have these same benefits.)

YOGURT

Called by some the weight-conscious person's best friend, yogurt (the unflavored non-fat version) can be used as a tasty substitute for almost any recipe calling for mayonnaise, sour cream, or even whipping cream. It is delicious mixed with fresh fruit and also works well in hot recipes. There are antibiotics in yogurt that have bacteria killing powers plus enzymes that "defuse" certain cancer causing chemicals.

MILK

Whether or not an adult needs or should have milk is a subject of some controversy among health authorities. However, there is growing evidence that skim milk does indeed have some benefits. Recent studies by the National Heart, Lung and Blood Institute indicate that men who drink skim milk are less likely to suffer from high blood pressure than non-milk drinkers.

TEA

Including tea in the super food category may come as somewhat of a surprise because of the negative publicity that caffeine has been receiving related to health. However, there is current research which indicates that ordinary tea (not the herbal varieties) can help prevent atherosclerosis and strengthen capillaries. Most Oriental societies (who also have low incidences of heart disease) have included this beverage in their diets for centuries and boast its digestive properties. Excessive tea drinking, however, can keep your body from absorbing iron, and too much caffeine can cause health problems for some individuals (including sleeplessness and elevated blood pressure).

AMERICAN CANCER SOCIETY "SUPER FOODS"

The American Cancer Society offers the following "Approved Shopping List" of foods which they suggest as a guideline to follow to help reduce the risk of some cancers.

- Strawberries, peaches, carrots, spinach and other vitamin A-rich foods

- Oranges, tomatoes, grapefruit, peppers and other foods high in vitamin C

- Cruciferous vegetables (broccoli, cauliflower, cabbage, Brussels sprouts)

- Chicken, fish and lean meats

- High-fiber fruits, vegetables and grains

- Low-fat dairy products

STRUCTURED FOOD PLAN

Although we present the basic concepts of several food plans, the details of the one you select and use should be developed by you. One of the reasons many people don't stick with a food plan long enough to lose the amount of weight they desire is because the food plans either don't fit their lifestyle or their food preferences. They become boring, lack sufficient variety, or they are too restrictive.

We have given a suggested version, The BALANCE Food Plan, at the end of this section. It is not necessary that you use this specific food plan. It is given as one alternative or approach in case you would like to use it. It is based upon a sensible, healthy approach to weight loss which incorporates good nutritional standards as well as taking into consideration dietary cholesterol guidelines. It is based upon approximately 1500 calories per day. If you choose to use the BALANCE food plan, it is not necessary to record daily calories, but you will need to weigh and measure food as well as record meals and snacks to make sure you are including all your nutritional requirements. It is important on any weight-loss plan to include the proper nutrients and to consume enough calories so you aren't sabotaging your basal metabolic rate.

We also recommend a multi-vitamin/mineral supplement taken either every day or every other day. Remember that vitamins work only in conjunction with food. Taken alone they pass through the body leaving no benefits for your system. For this reason, it works best to take them with meals. Please be aware that taking more than the recommended dosage can be dangerous and in some cases, fatal.

The important consideration with any food plan is that if you're starving your body nutritionally, no matter the numbers of calories you are consuming, then you are sabotaging your body's ability to stick to your plan and to achieve wellness. When using any food plan try to work with your body's natural rhythm. If you like and feel you need a big breakfast, then go lighter on lunch or dinner or snacks. If, on the other hand, your hungry time is in the evening, use your fruit for an evening snack or as dessert. We all have a different body rhythm. Working with it rather than trying to drastically change it will be more successful for you in the long run. Nothing in your life, including any food, is forbidden. You will find, however, if you don't already know, that some behaviors and some foods work better than others to allow you to achieve your goals! Learn to recognize these and use them. It's a choice you are free to make because you are the only one who is making up the rules here. Form a program you can live with!

Because this is your wellness plan it must be one that works well for you; that incorporates your lifestyle and tastes and eating patterns. Where a particular type of food plan will be successful for one person, it will be awkward or extremely unpleasant for another because of the structure and food choices. Let's face it, even though health experts suggest eating breakfast, for instance, there's a lot of leeway in what constitutes "breakfast". Some doctors and weight-loss plans suggest a high protein breakfast while others believe that complex carbohydrates (fruit and whole grain foods) tend to better quench hunger for a longer period. You will need to adjust your eating schedule and food choices to your needs. For some, that means only a mid-morning snack of fruit or a bran muffin; for others it means eating a larger meal earlier in the morning with no mid-meal snack. You will need to experiment to see which works best for you.

Our research has led us to what we believe are some of the best plans, and any one of them will work if followed. If you choose to use one of the plans we have listed as a guideline, that's fine. If you choose to modify or combine any of them so they will better fit your needs, this is also fine. Or, you can develop your own food plan using one of the models as a guide. We have listed suggested publications with each section that we consider to be excellent ones to give you details regarding the specific food plan. You may wish to purchase one of these publications or use one of your own choosing.

There are six basic systems that are currently popular:

Calorie counting

Food exchanges

Rotation plans

Nutrient counting

Combining plans

Psychological or behavior modifications plans

CALORIE COUNTING

Probably the most well known is the tried-and-true calorie counting system. With this type of plan you weigh and measure your food as well as keep track of the number of calories you consume each day, keeping calories within a set limit that you establish. If this system is used, we recommend 1400 to 1600 calories per day. Dropping below this amount may well adversely affect your basal metabolism rate (set point) and cause you to gain unwanted weight back quickly. (See section on "Set Point" for more detail.)

One key to sticking with a calorie-type plan is to use your daily caloric intake as a guideline on a day-today basis; but if needed, it can vary a bit as long as you stay within your total allotted calories per week. There may be situations where you have to go over the desired calories for one or two days during the week. This is preferable to saying, "what the hey, I've already gone over my limit, so I may just as well blow the rest of the week." What you should do is consider the overeating day (as long as it is within reasonable bounds) as allowable and make adjustment for it in a following day or two so that at the end of the week, you're still on target (based upon a week's total calories). If you build this into your plan, you won't feel you have failed if you have to exceed your desired calories one or two days. Many individuals tend to eat a little more on weekends, and if this seems to be a pattern you can't break, then use the first day or two following the weekend to cut back on calories so you will balance out for the week.

One thing you will need to watch closely if you chose this system is to make sure you include all the required food groups. See the "Eating Nutritionally" section for detail. If you nutritionally starve your body, even though are consuming an adequate amount of calories, you will eventually go off your food plan or suffer health problems. You will need to monitor your food plan closely to make sure your food intake is nutritionally sound. This also helps eliminate those terrible cravings we all get from time to time.

You may also find that you have better success by consuming your allowed calories in various ways. For instance, some individuals do better with six small meals a day. Others do fine with two larger meals. You may find that eating after eight o'clock at night keeps you from dropping off pounds even though you are within your calorie guides. For most people, three meals a day with a light snack to keep your blood sugar stabilized will work best. Your snack, if you choose one, should be a small fruit or vegetable serving. This provides both fiber and a small amount of fructose which will help keep your blood sugar from swinging from extreme lows to extreme highs, which is what happens when you eat too much refined sugar. If the blood sugar level is reasonably stable, you are much less likely to experience real hunger.

Each person's system, food preferences, eating patterns, and lifestyle differ. You will need to experiment to see which works best for you. We recommend that anyone using the BALANCE system use a calorie system for at least the first week of his wellness program in order to acquaint himself with the caloric value of foods. Daily food choices should include no more than 20% fat content, 60% to 70% complex carbohydrates (fruits, vegetables, whole grain products), and 10% to 20% protein. Most men tend to believe they need much more protein than they actually do. Current government recommended daily allowance (RDA) nutritional guidelines suggest that 4 to 6 ounces of protein per day is all we actually need. Remember, too, that protein also comes from vegetable sources as well as meat, fish, or poultry.

EXCHANGE PLANS

Using this system, you choose one or more items from each of several food group categories called "exchanges." (For instance, fruit exchange, bread exchange, vegetable exchange, protein exchange, etc.) You are allowed a specified number of "exchanges" from each group per day. The term "exchange" is used because a serving of food within a specific food category can be exchanged for another food within the same food group. This system is actually based upon calories (so many from each food group) and nutritional requirements, but it eliminates having to do your own calorie calculations. As with the calorie system, it is important to weigh and measure portions. This system helps make sure that you get the proper nutrition as well as eliminating the mathematics.

Most exchanges systems are based on a minimum of 1400 to 1600 calories per day for men. Weight Watchers, Diet Center, the Diabetes Association, and the Heart Association, among others, use an exchange system. *THE DIET CENTER PROGRAM* by Sybil Ferguson and any of the *WEIGHT WATCHERS* books are excellent sources that outline an exchange system as well as give recipes.

ROTATION SYSTEM

The rotation system is a variation of the calorie counting system, but you don't consume the same amount of calories each day. For instance, you eat 900 calories for three days, followed by 1500 for four days, then a week at 1800 calories, and then repeat the cycle. Advocates of this system feel it is more effective than the traditional calorie counting system. The definitive book on this subject is *THE ROTATION DIET* by Martin Katahn, Ph.D. (published by Norton & Co., New York). There is also a separate cookbook.

NUTRIENT COUNTING

Nutrient counting is not a new weight-loss concept. You may remember the carbohydrate counting fad during the 1970's where you kept track of the quantity of carbohydrates you ate daily rather than counting calories. The premise was that you could eat virtually all the protein and fat you wanted if you limited your carbohydrate intake to 60 grams or less per day. Many lost weight on this regimen, but in most cases, they put it back on almost immediately when they returned to a normal eating routine and their systems tried to stabilize. They also put their health at risk. The high protein diet was hard on kidneys, among other things, and like all fad-based weight-loss plans that aren't based upon sound nutrition, it proved to be a less that satisfactory solution to excess weight.

A more current version of nutrient counting focuses on eliminating dietary fat. Instead of counting calories or exchanges, this plan emphasizes counting only the grams of fat you eat. Theoretically, the amount of protein and complex carbohydrate calories won't affect your ability to lose weight (or maintain a desirable weight). This kind of eating is based upon a much more sound nutrition concept than those mentioned above, and it is potentially appealing because of the simplicity of keeping track of only one nutrient (fat) rather than counting everything you eat. Men should aim for 30 to 60 grams of fat per day, using half the total for breakfast and lunch combined, and half for dinner. It is important not to feel hungry, so complex carbohydrates are used freely as a means of appeasing your appetite. This is basically the same concept as several other weight-loss approaches that emphasize keeping your percentage of fat calories (or grams) between 10% to 30% of your total calories. However, I suspicion that you could follow the fat gram guidelines and still not lose weight if your total calories were excessive. Focusing on a nutritionally balanced food plan rather than focusing on only one nutrient has in most cases proved to be the most healthy and effective means of shedding pounds. Martin Katahn, Ph.D., also author of *THE ROTATION DIET*, explains this approach in detail in *THE T-FACTOR DIET*.

FOOD COMBINING

Food combining follows a school of thought that works for some, which is the concept that it is not what you eat, but how and when you eat it that causes overweight. For instance, it's all right to eat meat and potatoes, you just can't have them both at the same meal. Also, the time of day or the order in which you eat specific foods are also factors. Fruit, for example, must be eaten before meals (or as a meal), not after meals as we may be used to doing. If this system is of interest to you, and it appeals to many because it doesn't require calorie counting or restrictive portions, see *FIT FOR LIFE or FIT FOR LIFE II—LIVING HEALTH* by Harvey and Marilyn Diamond. The books contains concept, explanation, food plans, plus recipes.

PSYCHOLOGICAL OR BEHAVIOR MODIFICATION PLANS

One of the concepts behind the food plans using a psychological process is that if we are overweight, it may be because we have "programmed" ourselves into obesity. That is, we believe the reason we are fat is simply because we overeat, when the real cause may be that we overeat due to more complex reasons. This may seem a little hard to catch the first time around, so let's be a little more specific. As an example, if in your belief system there is some "payoff" for being overweight, then you will overeat. If you change the belief system, the fat will go away because you will eat differently once you are no longer "feeding" your problem. Obviously you must first subscribe to the interaction between mind and body in order for this kind of system to have relevance for you.

There are modifications and variations that have been very successful for individuals who could not lose weight, and keep it off, by focusing solely on their eating process. Self-hypnosis and the psycho-cybernetics approach are but two examples of this kind of approach. Using the power of the subconscious, you can reprogram your mind so that even though you may not consciously be aware of it, you will eat less and therefore lose weight. The key to success with this kind of plan is consistency and repetition; that is, the subconscious mind can be changed, but not overnight. It takes dedication and a specific regimen to accomplish weight-loss goals. In other words, our thoughts and feelings about ourselves are what keep us overweight. Our eating habits are a reflection of these attitudes.

If you are a compulsive eater, then there are some behavioral modification techniques that can be used to help you reprogram your behavior or to focus your compulsion into a positive addiction such as exercise. Most weight-loss plans today use some behavior modification techniques in conjunction with a specific food plan. We believe that to be successful with a weight-loss program you need to feel good about yourself, so we suggest that you consider using some of the techniques we have outlined. Please refer to the "Positive Power of the Mind" section. Excellent books that detail this approach are *DIETS DON'T WORK* by Bob Schwartz and his later book *DIETS STILL DON'T WORK,* as well as *THIN WITHIN* by Judy Wardell.

SUMMARY

There are successful dieters who have used and swear by one of the above systems over the others. As we stress again and again in the BALANCE program, there is not one perfect plan for everyone. What works for Bill may not work at all for Joe. You need to become knowledgeable about food, weight-loss techniques, exercise, and most of all yourself; then, using this workbook, structure your own plan. Perhaps the only thing your plan many have in common with Bill's plan is a mutual desire for wellness as well as the help and encouragement provided by your mutual involvement in a support group. You will have the same objective, but each of you will use different avenues of approach to reach it.

THE BALANCE PROGRAM FOOD PLAN

Approximately 1400 to 1600 Daily Calories

FOOD CATEGORY	1 SERVING EQUALS	TOTAL SERVINGS PER DAY
Dairy		2 servings
Non-fat milk	1 cup	
Plain yogurt (non-fat)	1 cup	
Cottage cheese (non-fat)	1/2 cup	
Protein	3 to 4 oz.	2 servings
Lean beef, veal, fish,		
Poultry (without skin)		
Eggs (limit to 4/week)		
Tofu (8 oz. = 3-1/2 oz. protein)		
Fruit		2 servings
fresh, canned or	1 medium fruit	
frozen without sugar	or 1 cup	
Vegetables	1 cup	3 servings
Green, yellow, leafy, etc.		
(non-starchy ones)		
Starch		4 servings
Uncooked cereal	1 ounce	
Cooked cereal	3/4 cup	
Rice, dried beans	1/2 cup	
Pasta	1/2 cup	
Bread	1 slice	
Potatoes, corn, etc.	1 medium	
Fat		1 tablespoon
Margarine or vegetable		
oils (monosaturated, i.e.		
canola or olive)		

Limit fat to 33 grams (approximately 300 calories)
Drink at least 8 to 10 glasses of water per day.
Drink no more than 1 to 2 cups caffeinated coffee per day.
Limit artificially sweetened sodas to 10 ounces per day.
Whenever possible, use fresh foods.
Use whole-grain rather than refined grain products.
By all means, use spices, herbs, and seasonings.
Limit sugar. Artificial sweeteners in moderation are all right.
No alcohol.
Take a daily multiple vitamin/mineral supplement.
OPTIONAL: One day per week, eat only fruit and vegetables (see "semi-fast" on page 172).

LEARN TO READ LABELS. COMMERCIALLY PREPARED FOODS USUALLY CONTAIN FATS AND SUGAR!

The Balance Program Food Plan provides all the necessary nutrients for well balanced eating. As mentioned earlier, it is a suggested food plan. You may wish to try a different regimen. We believe that calorie and nutrient awareness is an important element in your overall program. The Balance Program Food Plan stresses nutrients and serving sizes, rather than requiring you to keep track of calories. However, your caloric intake is an important consideration. If you eat the foods we have suggested in the amounts and portions stated, you will be eating from between 1400 and 1600 calories per day. If you eat too much (particularly foods with high fat content, i.e., those containing more than 30% of their calories from fat), you are not going to lose weight.

You will want to start focusing on getting your appetite under control as well as becoming aware of what kinds of food you are eating. High-fiber foods will help provide a feeling of fullness.

Learn to judge portion sizes. For instance, four ounces of meat, fish, or poultry is about the size of a deck of cards. Learn to judge how much you are eating by measuring and weighing as you begin your program. As you progress, you will become more proficient at knowing the size of a portion without weighing and measuring.

Try to have variation in what you eat. The boredom that sets in with eating the same food day after day is the undoing of many who are trying to lose weight. Take a scouting trip through the produce section of your grocery store. There is an amazing array of fruit and vegetables, many of which you may never have tried. Experiment with new foods that are healthy rather than focusing on having to give up foods that you love that contribute to your weight problem.

WEIGHING AND MEASURING FOOD

It is extremely important for you to learn to weigh and measure the food you eat. Both the calorie and the exchange system food plans are based on specific quantities. It's very difficult to estimate; the eye can be misleading. In all cases you need to measure and weigh portions, otherwise you are going to be overeating and wondering why you aren't losing weight.

As you get more competent at judging the size of food servings, you will better be able to judge the quantity of a restaurant meal. But, especially in the beginning of your program, try whenever possible to weigh and measure.

Buy a good food scale, available at drug, hardware or kitchen stores, and weigh your meat, fish, chicken, etc. Measure other items by volume.

EATING SMART

It will be to your great advantage to develop the ability to make smart food choices that will help rather than hinder your weight-loss process.

1. This means making sure you try to work with, rather than against, your body by choosing foods that meet your nutritional needs. For men, this may mean learning to reeducate your palate to some degree. If you come from the old "meat and potatoes school" and view salads as "rabbit food," you may have to do some work on your nutritional knowledge as well as your attitude. Meat is just fine, but more than likely you have been eating a great deal of fat along with it (both from the content of the meat itself as well as from the way it has been prepared) plus you probably have been eating much more of it than you actually need. Potatoes are a great food, but if you belong to the meat and potatoes school you generally add butter, gravy, and/or sauces that produce no nutritional benefits, but instead add unhealthy, high-cholesterol calories.

Salad may be rabbit food in your mind, but perhaps you've never tried the delicious combinations that can be had with a little imagination. Try adding a combination of chicken (or fish) with lettuce (all kinds plus other goodies such as green pepper, onions, celery, mushrooms, etc.) and a fruit (orange, or pineapple, for instance). You may find you are surprised by how delicious and filling a salad can be; and you now have the added benefit of a meal that works nutritionally with your body helping you to attain wellness as well as helping you to lose unwanted weight.

2. A calorie is a calorie, right? Not necessarily. Nutritionists now believe we burn up or process each of the food types differently. For example, fat calories are more likely to be stored as body fat than are calories from carbohydrates or protein. You burn more calories from eating carbohydrates than from eating protein or fat. Each of our bodies seems to have his own special way of assimilating food, and you may find you lose better eating one food rather than another—even though they have similar caloric values. As an example, you may lose easier eating fish and chicken than you do eating beef. Try listening to your body and watch closely to see what's going on. Six small meals may work better than three larger ones. Experiment to see what works best for you. Because each person's system is unique, what works for someone else may not work as well for you. You may not lose as well on foods that are "mushy" as you will on those that are more solid or dense (for instance a banana versus an apple). Most of us burn more calories if we eat food such as fruit and vegetables raw or lightly cooked rather than overcooked.

3. The final point to be aware of in order to eat smart is to educate yourself regarding lower calorie and lower fat equivalents. Sometimes the less fattening choice may even be just as tasty as the high calorie one. A bran muffin (homemade without all the excess sugar and fat) is a better choice than a croissant (as is a bagel). Become creative. If you crave a chocolate milkshake, instead try putting a quarter to half a cup of skim milk in a glass of sugarless chocolate pop. From a taste standpoint, it's not too bad a substitute, and you'll be saving over 300 calories. Add packaged seasoning mix to yogurt and use for vegetable dip, or put on your baked potato. Have the whole fruit instead of just the juice. The fiber will help make you feel fuller, and you'll have a health benefit from the fiber. Trim fat from meat before cooking. Consider combinations of food (non-fat stir fry, soups, or stews for instance). If you choose poultry, stick to the white portions because the dark meat has a higher fat content. Cooking poultry with the skin on, by the way, is all right. Just remember to remove the skin before eating. Do skin before cooking, however, for stir frying, soups, stews, etc. Instead of frying, try steaming, baking, or broiling. Use water, broth, wine or other non-fat liquid for stir frying. Lower fat versions of spreads (soft margarine) are generally considered to be a healthier choice than butter or solid margarine.

Get out your calorie counter and make up your own list of food equivalent choices so that the next time you have an urge to eat a "moderate food" you can substitute a "smart food" instead!

EATING SMART ACTIVITY

LOWER CALORIE EQUIVALENTS

Example:

INSTEAD OF:	CALORIES	SUBSTITUTE:	CALORIES	CAL. SAVED
Mayonnaise (1/4 cup)	400	Plain non-fat yogurt	28	372
French fries	300	Oven roasted "fries" or baked potato	100	200
Fried chicken (4-1/2 oz breast with skin)	350	Oven baked chicken breast (no skin)	140	210
Half & Half cream (2 TBL)	40	Skim milk (2 TBL)	11	29
Orange juice (1 cup)	112	Orange (whole)	64	48
Croissant	240	English muffin	130	110
Milkshake (1 cup)	260	Non-fat yogurt shake	140	120
Fruit pie (1 piece)	300	Apple, baked	95	205
Whole egg	75	Egg white	16	59
Cream-based soup	200	Broth-based soup	100	100
Milk, whole (1 cup)	150	Milk, skim	85	65

NOW MAKE A LIST USING YOUR OWN "SMART" CHOICES

WEIGHT-LOSS SUGGESTIONS

Always leave something on your plate.

Never eat while reading or watching TV.

Eat only when you are sitting down and when you are in a place that you have designated as an "eating place" (i.e., kitchen, dining room).

Eat small bites.

Eat slowly, putting fork down between bites, if necessary.

Really taste your food. Savor texture and flavor. Make every bite a sensory experience.

If you still feel hungry after you finish your allotted meal portions, try waiting for 20 minutes. It takes that long for your "appetite control monitor" to signal that you are full.

Try using a smaller plate.

To avoid temptation, plan your shopping list *before* you go to the market. Shop after meals. Don't ever shop when you are hungry. Try to buy all you need for several days.

Buy fresh fruit when it is in season and use water-pack or packaged-in-its-own-juice canned fruit if fresh isn't available.

Incorporate poultry (white meat) and fish into your daily meals rather than beef, if possible. If you do eat beef, try to limit it to once or twice a week.

Trim all visible fat from meat. You can cook poultry with the skin on, but remove before eating. All poultry, fish and meat should either be roasted, baked, broiled or poached. If you want to sauté, use a non-stick vegetable spray (PAM, for instance) or add a little beef, chicken broth, or water, if necessary, to keep food from sticking.

For items you would normally fry, such as eggs, use vegetable spray in a non-stick pan.

Try eating your vegetables raw part of the time for variety. When you do cook them, use a steamer basket and try leaving them a little crispy to maintain texture, flavor and nutrition.

To reduce your salt intake, try using herbs and spices, lemon juice, vinegar, mustard, etc. Catsup has a lot of both salt and sugar, so either eliminate or use sparingly. Soy sauce is all right, but in small quantities. (There is also a low-sodium soy sauce.)

Salad items should contain a wide variety of contents. For instance, there are many different kinds of lettuce as well as other greens such as spinach, bok choy, etc.

Vary these to keep your salads from getting monotonous. Also, raw cabbage, cauliflower, cucumber, green onions, tomatoes, radishes, zucchini, as well as bean and alfalfa sprouts may be used in almost unlimited quantities.

If you feel yourself getting too hungry between meals, particularly in the afternoon, allow yourself a low-calorie snack which will also keep you from overeating at dinner (a fresh fruit or vegetable is best).

Try to limit soda beverages. Most of these contain a lot of salt, but even those that are low sodium all contain a large amount of phosphorus which keeps your body from assimilating other vital nutrients. Also, some researchers claim that sodas (even the artificially sweetened ones) inhibit the weight loss process.

Eat a variety of foods. Include all the required food groups, but try to limit fat intake to not more than 20% of your total diet (preferably 10%). Most nutritionists today recognize the value of fiber (whole grains, fruits, vegetables, etc.) and recommend that at least 60% of your food come from this category. (Too much fiber, like too much of any one thing, however, can cause digestive problems. Balance is what is important.) This leaves about 20% to 30% of your food to be devoted to protein (including dairy products). A good balance of nutrients will help your system stabilize and will reduce food cravings that can turn into binges.

Protein, by the way, can be found in sources other than meat, fish or poultry. The chemical structure of protein is made up of a chain of 22 amino acids. Our bodies manufacture some of these amino acids, but nine of them must come from the food we eat. Without protein, necessary bodily functions cannot take place. Foods that contain these nine amino acids are called complete proteins (eggs, for instance). In general, all protein from animal sources is complete protein. Fruits, vegetables and grains contain only portions of the necessary amino acids, hence they are incomplete sources of protein. When combined properly, however, these incomplete sources can become complete proteins. In order to eat a complete protein, you need to *mix* or combine these sources. For instance, beans (or peas or lentils) plus rice make a complete protein. The beans have certain of the amino acids, while the rice has the others. Beans and brown bread (or corn bread) make a complete protein. Corn plus lima beans make a complete protein. While most men tend believe they need more, four to six ounces (about 56 grams or 224 calories) is nutritionally sufficient.

Meat, fish and poultry contain both protein and fat, so you need to take this into account when figuring out your nutrient quantities. As an example a 3-1/2 ounce trimmed portion of T-bone steak contains 10 grams of fat (90 calories) and 31 grams of protein (124 calories). The same portion of extra-lean ground been has 16 grams of fat (144 calories) and 28 grams of protein (112 calories). A 3-1/2 ounce piece of chicken breast, without skin, has 8 grams of fat (72 calories) and 31 grams of protein (125 calories). This is why, in most cases, poultry and fish are more desirable than beef for weight loss. If you plan to keep an exact record of the amounts of fat and protein you eat, you will want to get a reference guide that contains this information. However, it is not necessary to be this exacting, and most structured food plans (including the Balance food plan) simplify this for you.

Eliminate butter, fried foods, foods containing refined sugar and flour (cake, pie, cookies, etc.), bacon, luncheon meats, chips, nuts, ice cream, cream and coffee creamers, and cream cheese. Use non-fat milk rather than whole milk.

COOKING AND FOOD PREPARATION— LEARNING TO "COOK LIGHT"

One of the most important things to try to accomplish in your wellness program is eliminating foods that sabotage your health and weight goals. This means getting rid of the excessive and unhealthy fats and refined sugar you've been eating and using in your food preparation.

This doesn't mean you will never again feel full and satisfied or eat food that tastes delicious. Quite the contrary. Once you learn what you should be eating (including lots of fibrous foods that "sweep out" your system and help you feel full) and what you are better off without, the next step is learning how to prepare it. There are no "forbidden" or "bad" foods. However, there are some foods that you will come to believe are not healthy for you and that you will choose not to eat, (or at least to eat only in limited amounts). The next step is learning how to prepare delicious and satisfying meals and snacks. Because the results of this wellness plan are so effective for you, you will choose to continue eating in a healthy way for the rest of your life.

Almost any food that you would normally fry can be deliciously prepared without adding oil and without compromising flavor. Two of the most essential pieces of "working equipment" you will need are a non-stick fry pan and a vegetable steamer basket. Both are inexpensive and can be found in most hardware stores.

The first thing you should do as you start to prepare your meal is trim all visible fat from meat and poultry. Also remove the skin from poultry before eating, as this is where most of the fat is found. Boneless, skinless chicken breasts are best for a weight-loss plan, but other pieces are acceptable if skin is removed. By spraying the surface of your fry pan with a non-stick vegetable spray (such as PAM), you can successfully "fry" your food. Try adding a small amount of liquid (a couple of tablespoons, to start) if you have problems with sticking. Besides water, you can use bouillon or a little wine, or even lemon juice. Learn to "dry" fry or water sauté your fish, chicken, meat as well as veggies, or try combining them for a delicious stir-fry.

Another cooking technique is to use butter-flavored vegetable spray on food that you are baking in the oven. Potatoes are delicious this way. (Peel, cut into pieces; parboil for about 10 minutes, then bake at 400 degrees for about a half hour). Try wrapping fish, chicken and vegetables (separately or together) in foil to bake. With this technique you can add all kinds of spices and flavorings (taco seasoning, Cajun spice, etc.) as well as wine. Just sprinkle over your food, then seal in a foil packet and pop in the over for about a half hour at 400 degrees.

Learn to eliminate excessive sugar by substituting artificial sweeteners or use a natural source of sweetness such as frozen apple juice, applesauce, or bananas in your recipes. Note that EQUAL brand sweetener loses it sweetness under extended high-heat situations, so it cannot be used for baking. Any of the other sugar substitutes will work with baking, but if you use too much, your food will taste bitter. When using natural sweeteners such as sugar or honey, try reducing the amount called for in the recipe. (See section on "Sugar").

Unflavored non-fat yogurt can be used in most recipes calling for whipping cream, sour cream, or mayonnaise. Mixed in the blender with bleu cheese or a little Dijon mustard and sweetener (or moderate amount of honey), it makes an excellent salad dressing. Tofu is another food that can be used to make excellent desserts or used with vegetables for a stir-fry. When used for desserts, this soy derivative can be mixed in the blender with almost any fresh or frozen fruit (plus a little unflavored gelatin to thicken) to make a pudding-like concoction.

You may want to purchase one of the many excellent low-fat, low-calorie cookbooks on the market, or try experimenting and creating your own recipes. LEARN TO "COOK LIGHT".

EATING OUT

Your food plan need not prohibit eating in restaurants or eating at someone else's home. A restaurant meal can provide variety and a boost to your motivational process. It can keep you from feeling deprived. Armed with the knowledge of what you can eat and how it should be prepared, you can choose delicious, allowable foods that fit within your food program. Try to choose restaurants that offer the kinds of food and cooking that work with your wellness program. This may take a little research on your part, but it will be worth it. Also, because such a large segment of our population is concerned with health, most restaurants can accommodate special dietary requirements when requested. Ask that food be served without butter or sauces; avoid fried foods or foods high in sugar content.

At lunch, for instance, a wide variety of salads is available in most restaurants. Simply choose one that incorporates your allowable food plan choices, then add your own dressing or have dressing on the side and use sparingly. Lemon juice or vinegar, without the oil or with a small amount of oil (no more than one tablespoon per day), is also an excellent choice. If you do have salad, try to make sure that it includes some source of protein, otherwise you will probably be overly hunger at dinnertime and tend to overeat.

Lean meat (broiled) along with some cottage cheese is all right as is steamed or roasted fish or chicken. Watch out for the skin on chicken, because that is where most of the fat is. Omelets are also a good choice if you don't have to watch cholesterol levels. (The American Heart Association suggests limiting eggs to four a week.) Cottage cheese and fresh fruit is another good choice.

If you are going to eat dinner out, and you will either be eating late or may have some limited food choices available, try eating an apple beforehand. Apples seem to have some mysterious ability to help satisfy hunger, and because of their natural fructose content, help stabilize your blood sugar levels. (See section on Fat and Sugar for more detail.)

HOW TO HANDLE FOOD CRAVINGS

1. Go through the "Is Food What I Really Want" activity to make sure the specific food you are craving is really what you went.

    A   Do you really want it, or is it an old habit?

    B. Is the craving the result of a temporary stimulus (i.e., you walked past a chocolate chip cookie stand or saw French fries advertised on television)?

2. Try an activity from your "Instead of Eating" list and see if the craving goes away.

3. Have a small (a few bites) portion of whatever it is you think you can't live without. THIS ONLY WORKS FOR SOME AND CAN BOOMERANG ON OTHERS, SO USE DISCRIMINATION, PLEASE! FOR SOME, A BITE OR TWO ENDS UP CAUSING AN OVEREATING OR BINGE REACTION.

4. Make a substitution for something else you like that has fewer calories or that has less fat and/or sugar content; i.e., instead of ice cream, try a frozen banana or mix non-fat yogurt with fresh fruit. Instead of a croissant, eat half an English muffin. (See "Eating Smart Activity - fewer Calorie Equivalents".)

5. If you do decide you really must have what you're craving, go ahead and eat it — but don't overeat! DON'T BINGE! The name of the game is BALANCE. Nothing is forbidden; you are learning to reeducate your appetite so that you want to choose foods that are healthy for you. Remember that too much sugar and fat aren't healthy; those are the culprits that caused your overeating problems, so try to avoid them.

6. Do a "make-up" day. If you really must eat "it", then cut back on your food on the following day or two to compensate for your extravagance.

IV

USING THE POSITIVE POWER OF THE MIND

USING THE POSITIVE POWER
OF THE MIND

The important objective in the BALANCE program is achieving and maintaining good health, which means wellness and balance in mind, body and spirit. Taking off excess weight is, of course, a primary activity in achieving this goal. But keeping it off is the real key to your physical well-being.

This is why we are opposed to programs that promise quick weight loss through a liquid-only regimen or by eating pre-measured, packaged foods. These kinds of programs will cause you to lose weight, but they won't help you learn how to choose, shop and cook the foods that will keep off those pounds. These kinds of food plans force an unnatural, and many times unhealthy, eating regimen on you that can trigger binges or weight fluctuations that make weight maintenance nearly impossible. In addition, there is a possibility that if you lose weight too quickly you may develop gallstones which can require removal of your gall bladder. Over the long haul, drinking liquid diet meals or eating only packaged diet clinic foods neither reeducates your palate nor helps you change old eating patterns. Eating is a physical necessity; overeating or eating foods that cause poor health is not. This latter kind of eating is a habit that can be changed. This is why behavior/response modification (helping you change old habits that don't work) is such an important part of the BALANCE concept.

First, let's describe what this means as it relates to you. Weight loss and weight maintenance do not have to be synonymous with everlasting denial of everything you love to eat. They do not mean continual deprivation. It means learning some new ideas and techniques that will help you replace old habits and the "old tapes" that are now going around in your mind. This mental process will help bring about the physical changes you are seeking: changes that include bringing youth and wellness back into your life to stay.

Your mind is a marvelously complex source of thought and feeling that might be compared to an iceberg. The thinking, acting portion we are aware of is like the part of the iceberg that we are able to see above water. This is the conscious mind, which includes both emotional and intellectual capabilities. There is a very large portion of our mind, however, that is like the part of the iceberg that is underwater. This is the subconscious (or some use the term unconscious) portion of the mind. It's there, but we are not always aware of its existence because it's not as easy to access. This doesn't mean that we have two separate minds operating within us. It's just a convenient terminology or point of reference to simplify our understanding of the simultaneous, dual functions that go on within us: one is obvious and direct, the other is much more subtle.

Most individuals who are chronically overweight have a problem that is not just about food. As you have seen from our chart on "Conditions that Contribute to Overweight," we have listed 14 possible reasons that might have some bearing on your weight problem. For most of us, there are a combination of reasons or multiple causes with one common result: obesity that is a threat to our health. If being overweight is about more than food, then, it only makes sense to try and (1) find out what these impacts are, and (2) see how we can change them.

As we have pointed out again and again, each of us is unique. This is why some of the activities may work better than others for you.

What we are offering are some techniques that have been tried in the past by many others and that have worked. They are "helpers" to get you from where you are now on to where you want to be. You won't know if they work if you don't give them a try.

It is our firm belief that in addition to changing your eating habits and participating in an exercise program, you will have better success in reaching your wellness goals if you also use the positive power of your mind to help you. These techniques include:

- focused relaxation

- visualization (mental imagery)

- affirmations

Using one or all of these techniques are aids that can help you change your eating behavior through the use of your subconscious mind. The key to success using these techniques is regularity and repetition. The subconscious mind can be "reprogrammed," and old tapes can be replaced with new ones that you create to allow you to achieve and maintain your wellness goals.

Changes won't come overnight. They will be gradual, and they will be dependent on your underlying motives. If you are resistant to the idea of losing weight, it will be more difficult. You must make and keep your commitment to use these techniques in order for them to be of value to you.

Emotional or compulsive overeating is a response to something that's going on in your life and in your mind. If you can change your reaction to whatever is stimulating you to overeat, then you will change the behavior (or response). Through the use of the worksheet activities, you will be able to identify the "triggers" and the subconscious beliefs that cause you to overeat. Then, using the suggested modification techniques, you can gradually change to a response that is more appropriate.

If you do not choose to do these activities, it's up to you, but we urge you to at least learn a relaxation technique to help you counteract the negative effects of stress that may come as part of a weight-loss program or that may already exist in your life. Each of us encounters stress, and a focused relaxation technique has been found to be a crucial aid in keeping our systems (mental, physical and spiritual) in balance. Your relaxation technique (described in detail in the following pages) can be done as a religious prayer or without a spiritual element, whichever works better for you. We hope you will develop a "positive addiction" to this form of helping your mind and your body.

FOCUSED RELAXATION

Learning to use a focused relaxation technique is an important part of a wellness program. It's a method by which you can help your mind and your body counteract daily stress, and it can help you modify behaviors that have contributed in the past to your overeating problem. Using a focused relaxation technique can also play a major role in making and keeping your body healthy.

We use the term "focused relaxation" to encompass a process that has been used for centuries in almost every culture and that goes by many names. We suggest you not focus on the terminology, but rather on the process. Among the terms used for what is basically the same elementary principle is prayer, meditation, inner silence, biofeedback, self hypnosis, auto suggestion, and even daydreaming. No matter what term you choose, it is a method of "shifting" your mental gears and putting yourself in neutral for a short time. It is a method you can use to access your subconscious mind in order to help enhance your overall health or to bring about a heightened sense of well-being. It produces a unique state of rest that is particularly beneficial to involuntary body functions.

In order to achieve the most benefit from this process, it is necessary for you to do it on a regular basis. As you get more used to whatever technique you choose, you will find it easier to become physically and mentally relaxed, and to enjoy the wellness benefits that come about as a result of these short sessions.

First you will need to choose a specific body or muscle relaxing technique, and then you will need to decide what you want to accomplish once you have made your subconscious mind receptive.

To begin, you will need to set aside at least one, and preferably two short periods every day (say, one first thing in the morning, and one in the evening). A fifteen-to twenty-minute session is usually sufficient if you do it regularly. You are training your conscious mind and your body to totally relax, and the more often you practice, the easier it will be to reach this level of relaxation and the better will be the results you are seeking.

Sit in a comfortable chair or lie down. Some individuals find they tend to fall asleep when the are totally prone, so you will need to decide which works better for you. Make sure your clothing is loose and comfortable. Try to find a setting that is free from noise and distractions. Sometimes soft background music helps provide a desirable atmosphere.

Next try to free your mind from all the things you may have been thinking or worrying about, and begin to concentrate on relaxing your muscle groups. Start by taking three deep cleansing breaths. Hold each one for a few seconds, then let it out slowly. Try to allow your body to become limp and free from muscle tension. To do this, begin at your feet and move gradually up toward your head, or you can reverse the process and start at the top. Some individuals, particularly until they get adept, find that recording their suggestions on a tape and playing them back works better than trying to do the process silently. As you start to relax, make sure your body is comfortable, and then think about your feet (if you decide to start at that end). Picture your feet in your mind, and make a conscious effort to relax all the muscles in your feet, then slowly move on up to your calves. Continue to breathe deeply and slowly. Visualize and relax those muscles. You may want to tighten and then relax the tension in each area as you proceed. Now let this relaxed feeling continue up your thighs, up the abdomen, across your shoulders and down your arms, then continue up the neck and head. Suggest to yourself that you are now totally relaxed and free from all tension. You might want to use a specific code phrase or some code words such as "calm and relaxed" etc., so that as you continue to practice you can very quickly reach the desired state of relaxation by using the code word shortcut rather than going through the whole process. Slow breathing is important to the process, so be sure you take long, deep breaths. With regular practice, your body can very quickly achieve a state of total relaxation.

In addition to the muscle relaxing method, there are other formulas you can choose, such as the elevator method where you let your body become more and more relaxed as you ride from the tenth floor down to the first floor. See yourself sitting in a comfortable chair in the elevator, and as you go down each floor, tell yourself that you are becoming more comfortable and more limp until, as you reach the ground floor, you are totally relaxed.

Another method that works well is counting backwards. Starting with ten, tell yourself that you are relaxed and comfortable, then continue with the process counting nine, eight, etc., until you reach one, when you will be totally relaxed. Again, deep breathing is part of the relaxing process.

Don't worry that you will not be able to "reawaken" yourself. You are always in control, and the most extreme thing that can happen to you when you are using one of these techniques is that you will fall into a normal sleep from which you will awake just as you would any other time you were catching a short nap.

Once you have achieved a state of physical and mental relaxation, it is time for you to let your mind take over and begin to focus on your objective. Use this focused state of concentration to make suggestions such as the affirmations you have chosen. Remember to think in terms of present tense. Use this short time to picture yourself in a body that is fit and healthy. See yourself looking exactly the way you would like to look. You may want to take a short walk to a lovely meadow or to the ocean beach or to fly through the clouds. As you do these mental activities, your physical body will be reaping the maximum benefits in terms of wellness. This state is even called the "healing silence" by many. Focused relaxation can also be used to promote health benefits such as controlling pain and reducing high blood pressure.

If you find you are becoming distracted and you are starting to think about other things, pull back your concentration by taking a deep breath and silently repeat your code words (i.e., calm and relaxed or whatever). Especially as you first begin, it's easy for the mind to wander. Your ability to focus and concentrate will improve with practice.

After you are ready to come back to your normal way of thinking, you can use a counting method to suggest to yourself that as you say the number five you will begin to feel energy returning to your body. As you continue to count down from four to three, two and then one, suggest that you will feel wide awake, refreshed, and that all discomforts serving no purpose will have left your body. Now stand up, take another deep breath, let it out slowly, and stretch.

If you choose this technique for prayer or spiritual meditation, use this time to ask for help and guidance in attaining your wellness goals. Whichever method you choose, you will find this is a marvelous way to relieve tension and stress and to bring about well-being.

VISUALIZATION (IMAGING)

Visualization, or the process of mental imaging, should be used along with your chosen relaxation technique. Tapping the power of your unconscious and using your imagination will aid you in achieving your weight-loss goal. There are even recent studies that demonstrate you can achieve better results with strengthening and stretching your muscle groups if you visualize them at the same time you are exercising. Though scientists are not sure exactly how or why the process works, there is enough evidence collected to give credence to the concept of mental imaging.

Visualization can help you relieve stress, strengthen your motivation, as well as improve your mental and physical health. We all daydream from time to time, and that's actually what visualization is all about. The only difference is that now you are going to direct your mental energy toward helping you achieve a specific goal.

First you need to be in a quiet setting where there are no distractions or noise. You will need only about fifteen minutes for a session. (We suggest two or more sessions per day.) Relax your body using whatever relaxation technique you have chosen. Once you feel you are completely relaxed, try to form a precise, clear picture in your mind. The picture could be a meadow full of flowers, a shady forest glen, a mountain top, or you could see yourself walking or relaxing on the beach. Create a safe, pleasant, vividly colored scene. Try to hear the sounds of nature (the birds, the ocean, etc.) and then once you have the scene fixed in your mind, picture yourself in this scene just as you would like to look: trim, fit, virile, youthful, filled with vitality and good health. See yourself from several angles. Appreciate how well you look. See yourself enjoying happiness and well-being. Hold the picture for several minutes, then allow yourself to come back to your normal way of thinking and "reawaken" your physical energy. You may also want to visualize yourself eating and enjoying healthy, non-fattening foods or actually refusing those foods which you know will sabotage your weight-loss efforts. See yourself feeling full and satisfied without overeating.

Don't get hung up on the terminology and don't worry if at first you don't "see" anything, or if your mind wanders. It takes practice to achieve competence and results with this technique. The process will become more comfortable and effective with regular use.

CAR ACTIVITY

In your mind, picture the ultimate car of your dreams. This is a fantasy where the only limits are those you establish. It can be an actual car or one you create. How big is it? How much power does the engine have? How do the gears work? What color is it? Picture the finely tuned piece of machinery as you are traveling through a beautiful countryside.

Because your car is such a magnificent piece of machinery, you always give it the best of care: the best fuel and maintenance; your best driving skills. You never drive it beyond its limits. You would never intentionally harm your fantasy car... because the catch is, this is the only car you will ever have. It must last you the rest of your life.

Now imagine that same car is your body. Do you give yourself the best or do you abuse your "machinery?" From now on, begin to view your body as a magnificent piece of equipment. Treat it with respect. Give it only the best fuel. Never intentionally abuse it. Stop and think about what you are doing to the machine that is you when you over consume food or drink. Consider what happens inside your machine when your engine boils over with anxiety, anger, fear or guilt.

Make a commitment to yourself that you will treat your body in the best way possible...because it's the only one you will ever have, and you deserve the best!

AFFIRMATIONS

Our bodies obey instructions from the mind. If we change our minds (attitudes, feelings, beliefs, etc.), then our behavior and the way it affects our bodies also changes. One behavior that can be changed is the overeating that causes us to be unwell.

Affirmations are a tool that can be used for this kind of behavior/response modification. The basic principle behind the theory of using affirmations is the idea that certain subconscious portions of the mind which control some of our behavior and attitudes can be "programmed" for change. If we use a correlation here, we could compare the brain to a computer with the subconscious mind operating as a software program. Quite simply, affirmations are words or phrases or sentences we repeat over and over (usually aloud, but they can also be done silently). Research indicates that for many individuals, the repeated use of a specific phrase can help change certain behaviors and attitudes. However, deeply held values are very difficult to change once we become adults.

Affirmation techniques are currently being successfully used in many well-known business and self-help programs as well as for weight loss. The use of affirmations can be a key step in changing attitudes you have about yourselves that influence your weight. This technique seems to work better for some than for others. If, for instance, you don't really believe that what you're trying to affirm is possible, then your belief system is going to win out in the long run.

As an example, you can tell yourself that you are successful, lovable, handsome, or whatever you want. But if your underlying belief is that you are not capable of becoming those things, then tacking words on your wall, your mirror, or your refrigerator and looking at them when you shave, or writing them twenty times a day, or saying them over and over again, is probably not going to help you. If you have some strong underlying belief that tells you that you are not entitled to be successful, for instance, then affirmations by themselves will probably not change this for you. You need, first, to find out why you believe you are unworthy of being successful (or lovable or trim), and then change that belief to a more positive one that works better for you. So to say that affirmations do work or do not work is not a clear-cut situation. It is not necessarily that simplistic. To a great extent, it depends upon your mind set. Many individuals have had successful results using affirmation techniques. Why not give it a try? What have you got to lose (pun intended!)?

As they apply to weight loss, you will need to work out for yourself what your affirmations are going to be and then use them regularly as a form of autosuggestion. The key word here is regularly. Changing attitudes or habits is much like learning to play tennis. It is the repetition of going through the motions over and over again that finally pays off. Behavioral scientists believe it takes at least 21 days of "programming" for change to begin to take place. Figuratively speaking, you are erasing old tapes and replacing them with new ones.

One of the affirmations that has been widely used and that has been around for many years is "each and every day, in every way, I'm getting better and better." This may be a good one to use in conjunction with others you are going to incorporate. As you keep inputting these thoughts into your mind, soon you will begin to see the results as you begin to look and feel better. You will be losing weight and you will be healthier.

This phenomenon is something that's not totally understood, but the process of actually verbalizing these statements helps implement them into our brain which operates like a computer to run our bodies. Affirmations can work, and they can help motivate you to lose weight and feel better.

What you will be trying to accomplish is changing negative or destructive feelings and responses to positive feelings and responses; reinforcing and enhancing self esteem and an "I'm okay" attitude. Each of us has value an individual; not all of us believe it. That is one of the many reasons why some of us have weight problems. Affirmations can be a positive key to helping solve this problem.

Keeping in mind that affirmations are not a cure all, but rather a tool we are using with this program, we have listed some suggested affirmations. You will need to develop a set that specifically works for you. The ones we have listed are merely to give you an idea of what we are talking about. Ideally, you should say your affirmations several times a day. To begin with, keep your list fairly short. Try to focus on one thing at a time. You will probably want to change or modify your affirmations as you progress or better refine your understanding of your problem areas or areas in your life that you want to improve.

GUIDELINES FOR WRITING AFFIRMATIONS

1. You must have a strong motivation that relates to the affirmation. You must really want what you are trying to affirm.

2. Your affirmation must be phrased in positive language. For instance, instead of saying "I won't eat too much," say, "I only eat as much as I physically need." Instead of "I am not hungry," use "I am full and satisfied."

3. Use present, not past or future tense. Instead of saying, "I am going to be fit and handsome," say "I am fit and handsome." Remember that what you are trying to do here is reprogram the subconscious mind. Research indicates this process works best when we suggest that the desired change is already in effect.

4. Use specific affirmations and work on one thing at a time until you feel you are ready to progress to another area.

5. Be aware of emotionally loaded words. Be carefully to phrase your suggestions so that they are not words that trigger unpleasant emotions or anxiety for you (like the word diet, for instance).

6. Use language that triggers your imagination, even though it may seem to be exaggerated.

7. Make a commitment to say your affirmations at least ten times each day. Repetition is the key to success with this tool.

8. For some affirmations, a time limit or target date works well. For instance you could say, "By (name a date) I weigh (name an amount). Make the time and weight ones that are within reason. Notice the suggestion is not "will weigh." You want your statements in present tense.

9. Use short sentences with simple language, at least at the beginning of this process. If you choose to use a longer, more complex statement, then limit your number of affirmations to one or two.

10. As you progress, you will probably want to add to or refine your affirmations.

SUGGESTED AFFIRMATIONS

Below are some suggested affirmations. You will want to develop your own list. Perhaps you will need to experiment a little to find those that work best for you. You may want to write your affirmations out several times a day, or just say them aloud. Try putting them on a small file card so you can carry them with you.

THIS WELLNESS PROGRAM WORKS FOR ME.

IT IS EASY FOR ME TO LOSE WEIGHT.

I LOVE AND APPRECIATE MYSELF.

I LET GO OF ALL NEGATIVE SELF IMAGES AND ATTITUDES.

THE MORE I APPRECIATE MYSELF, THE HEALTHIER I AM.

BECAUSE I DESERVE THE BEST, I ONLY EAT WHAT IS HEALTHY FOR MY BODY. I THINK AND ACT LIKE A SLIM PERSON.

I LOSE WEIGHT BY THE POWER OF MY MIND (OR HIGHER POWER SOURCE).

I USE MY MIND TO CREATE WELLNESS IN MY BODY.

I DESERVE WELLNESS.

I KNOW THE DIFFERENCE BETWEEN PHYSICAL AND PSYCHOLOGICAL HUNGER.

I EAT ONLY UNTIL I AM PHYSICALLY SATISFIED.

I CONTROL MY APPETITE.

EVERY DAY, IN EVERY WAY, I'M GETTING BETTER AND BETTER.

EATING AFFIRMATION

Read these three sentences aloud before each meal and/or snack. Stop for a few seconds to reflect on what they mean, then continue with your meal.

1. Eating is not what makes me overweight. Overeating and eating the wrong foods is what makes me overweight.

2. I can choose what I eat, and I choose to eat only that food which brings me wellness.

3. I can choose how much I eat. I choose to eat only as much as my body needs to maintain a state of wellness.

SABOTAGE

Sabotage seems to be a negative word that dredges up images that are less than pleasant. However, we would be remiss if we didn't bring to your attention how the actions and reactions of others can influence your success with this program. You need to be aware of these potential situations so that you can leap over the hurdles they present. You also need to be alert for actions of your own that put unnecessary obstacles in your wellness path.

Some sabotage is deliberate, some not. Some is very subtle, some quite obvious. If you understand the motives that lay beneath, however, you may be better able to immunize yourself against the effects.

Let's take a look at some specifics. You're working hard on getting your health act together, but your best buddy still overindulges and looks like a Sumo wrestler. He razzes you about your involvement with the program and tries to persuade you with reasoning such as, "What the hell, come on, let's go have a few brews. A couple won't hurt, and you look great just the way you are. Don't be a wet blanket!"

What's happening with your friend here is not about you so much as it is about himself. Misery loves company. He doesn't want you to be slim and trim if it makes him look bad. If he lacks the incentive to take good care of himself, he doesn't need your dedication to wellness to act as a mirror where he will be forced to view his own image. If he is really your friend, he'll respect your desire to get and stay healthy.

Wives or lovers can often be intimidated and experience feelings of insecurity when they see their partners involved with a weight-loss program. Although they may not be exactly aware of what's bothering them, they may subconsciously feel they will be rejected if they don't measure up as perfect physical specimens. Or they may anguish over the possibility of abandonment. If you're trying so hard to look and feel good, they may worry that you're going to dump them for a younger and/or spiffier version. As we have said, this can be done very subtly with, "Oh, come on, a little bit won't hurt. Don't be so rigid," etc. That's why in some cases you will need to be in control of your meal planning, shopping and cooking. For some of you this will be the case; for others, your wives will be your greatest ally. If your partner does seem to have feelings of anxiety about your program, what she needs at this time is extra love, patience, and reassurance. Special tenderness in the form of touching and talking it out will usually help. Try to share your feelings with each other.

The other area you need to be watchful for is self-sabotage. Remember the story about the fellow whose arm hurt every time he bent it? He went to the doctor and demonstrated how every time he bent his arm, it caused him pain. To this the doctor replied, "Well, if it hurts when you do that, then don't do that." Obviously, real physical pain isn't something you should ignore.

What we're trying to illustrate is that if you know you have a particular situation that triggers overeating, then try to avoid that particular thing until it no longer presents an irresistable temptation. If there's a special restaurant where you can't eat without having their triple-decker super dessert, save that experience until you are on maintenance or as a special reward for a major goal achievement. If watching TV food commercials triggers your eating response mechanism, get up and leave the room when they are airing. When the imagination and will power are put into conflict, the imagination is going to win. That's why imagining yourself as a thin person has positive results.

Don't deliberately place temptation in your path. Substitute something less threatening that you might find just as pleasurable: hobbies, exercise, group involvement, etc.

Share potential sabotage experiences with your support group and your wellness partner. Give and receive advice an how to handle such situations.

SABOTAGE ACTIVITY

1. What are ways my spouse/lover tries to sabotage my wellness goals?

2. How can I reassure her or explain my concerns so that she becomes more supportive?

3. How do my friends (business associates, etc.,) pose a threat to my wellness goals?

4. How can I work this out with him (them) so the sabotage behavior is neutralized?

5. What "events" (occasions, environments, activities, etc.) tend to trigger my tendency to overeat?

6. Which of these events above can I either eliminate or modify so they no longer pose a potential threat to my wellness plan?

STRESS

We are hearing and reading a lot about stress these days. It's a popular topic for seminars, articles, books and conversation plus what increasingly seems to be a catch-all term for everything that ails us. This is certainly not inappropriate because stress (or more to the point how we handle stress) can be an important factor in our lives. It is estimated that at least 70% of the physical problems doctors see are stress related.

However, as with many of the phases we Americans seem to go through, all this emphasis on stress may also tend to help us develop attitudes and make excuses for ourselves that are not necessarily to our benefit. What we may have taken for granted in some years past as part of life's normal ups and downs, we may now focus upon more intently allowing ourselves to feel we are entitled to "rewards" (such as excess food, alcohol and drugs) because of "all that stress we are under." The point here is two-fold. First, it's not stress per se that is our problem. It's how we choose to handle it. And second, because stress is an inherent part of life, it's the *degree* to which we are subjected to it that has an impact upon our overall well-being.

According to the late Dr. Hans Selye who pioneered stress research and who is still credited as being the definitive authority on the subject, "stress is the spice of life." We've come to believe that stress is that deadly thing that kills us. According to Dr. Selye, however, "stress is not something to be avoided." Stress is a fact of life, and it can be either pleasant or unpleasant. More to the point, what we should try to avoid or control is distress.

Simply eliminating negative experiences from your life will not eliminate undesirable stress results. Developing and improving the positive aspects of your life is what seems to be more important to mental and physical well-being. Interestingly, current research also indicates that the kind of stress that raises blood pressure and poses a threat to health in general is not from the major traumas or misfortunes we encounter such as job loss, divorce, etc. What seems to do the most damage are the "little things" that get to us such as driving in heavily congested traffic, arguments at home or at work, etc. Even though these kinds of hassles are for the most part unavoidable, we can learn to handle them in such a way that they have the least possible adverse effect on our health.

A certain amount of stress (and again, it's the balance that counts) is actually healthy. Loneliness, boredom, feelings of futility and helplessness all seem to be much more devastating to our physical systems than the stimulating kinds of stress that we generally identify as distressing. One man's "stress" is another man's stimulation or challenge. What is viewed as a problem for one person may be viewed as an opportunity by someone else. In general terms, stress is only a problem if you choose or allow yourself to make it one. Even then, it's a matter of degree. The glass can be half empty or half full.

Hard work, for instance, is not necessarily stress producing. Your perception of your degree of control over a situation is a much better indicator of what will probably be stress producing for you. If you are involved in a situation where you believe you can exercise some degree of control in the outcome, you are going to be much less likely to experience harmful stress than in situations where you feel you are the victim.

It is possible to adapt your response to what you perceive as a stressful situation. The type, frequency, duration, and intensity of the stress are all factors, of course. We need a certain amount of stimulation, but too much over stimulation can be stress producing. We need a certain amount of tranquillity in our lives, but boredom can be stress producing. Your ability to be mentally flexible is one of your best defenses against the effects of harmful stress.

Stress responses can be compared from an external and an internal viewpoint or from a cause and effect viewpoint. For example, causes of stress can be arguments, boredom, excitement or dissatisfaction with life; effects can be illness, pain or changes in our lives that are brought about as the result of the "causes." When the body encounters what it determines is stress, we respond with an internal "fight or flight" mechanism. Our body undergoes a biochemical response and starts pumping out adrenaline or other hormones and chemicals. These "internal" responses can then take the "external" form of muscular tension, increased heart rate, accelerated breathing, sweating, anxiety, constant fatigue, excessive eating or drinking, frequent colds and headaches. Prolonged, these symptoms can affect aging, health, and resistance to disease. Chronic stress can cause exhaustion, high cholesterol levels, plugged arteries, heart damage, joint inflammation and ulcers, to name but a few.

Typical emotions that trigger the stress response include fear, guilt, aggravation, joy/elation, harassment, challenge, concern over what others think of you, manipulation, humiliation, embarrassment, and lack of quality time alone. The list could go on.

There are techniques you can use to change or modify your stress responses. Rather than literally feeding your stress with food, learn to use some alternative methods:

- The one that has had the best success is learning to use a focused relaxation technique.

- Create a mental "safe place" and go there for a few minutes when you get overly tense.

- Practice deep breathing by first emptying your lungs of air, then slowly filling them up (taking ten or more seconds), and finally exhaling, letting shoulders and chest drop and relax.

- Exercise—even a short walk can do wonders.

- Take a long, relaxed bath or shower; water seems to be very therapeutic.

Without some degree of stress, life would be exceedingly bland. We humans are problem solvers; some of us just seem to create or encounter more problems than others. However, it's not our stress that is killing us; it's our *reaction* to the stress.

STRESS AND ITS RELATIONSHIP TO OVEREATING

Pressure, whether from your business or personal life, often results in the kind of stress that increases your desire to overeat. One of the most common responses to stress is the compulsion to overeat. In fact, this problem is now so prevalent that it is classified as an eating disorder.

There are several possible motivations that make us want to eat to relieve stress. For some chronic overeaters, any unpleasant feeling is interpreted as hunger. This includes such feelings as tension, depression, anxiety, and even anger. The psychological or emotional hunger takes the form of food cravings that are much more powerful than physical or real hunger. Eating to relieve or appease these emotional hungers, unfortunately, only provides short-term relief or satisfaction. The eating only distracts you from what is really bothering you. Binge eating is the result of not dealing constructively with other problems in your life. What you need to do is identify the cause of these emotions and find a more satisfactory way of dealing with them.

We've all been conditioned to respond to eating as a source of relaxation, comfort and being nurtured. From a strictly chemical point of view, eating certain foods actually can provide or stimulate our bodies to produce calming substances. We develop a learned or conditioned response to using food to calm ourselves. This is why behavior/response modification techniques can help by showing you ways other than eating that will work to help you relax or feel less anxious.

For some of us, emotional tension produces an increase in muscular tension. We actually store stress in the form of tense muscles, and the act of chewing can help relax this tenseness.

When we are relaxed, we have a natural reserve of energy and are less likely to seek food than when we are over stressed. Stress responses differ greatly from person to person. What can cause you to experience a great amount of anxiety can produce excitement or stimulation in someone else. It's a matter of degree and your individual response, not the situation itself, that needs to be addressed. Boredom, for instance, can trigger some of us to overeat, while it has the opposite effect on others.

To effectively combat stress, it is recommended that you incorporate a relaxation technique into your wellness program. It is important to use whatever technique you choose on a regular basis. The kind of relaxation we are talking about doesn't mean participating in or watching sports, television, or going on vacation. Those may be relaxing for you, but they also stimulate you. You need to incorporate a mental relaxation technique into your life that will help you better handle the stress that causes you to overeat.

20 STEPS FOR MANAGING STRESS

1. Use a focused relaxation technique on a daily basis.

2. Take some time every day, if only for a few minutes, to spend some quality time alone.

3. Get at least 30 minutes of aerobic-type exercise a minimum of three times a week.

4. If you smoke—quit! If you drink, limit alcohol to not more than 1-1/2 ounces per day. Limit coffee to two or three cups a day.

5. If you feel tense, anxious, hostile, etc., go ahead and express your feelings. Don't put them in your "gunnysack" and pack them around. Clear the air, but do it in a constructive, rational manner.

6. Avoid, if possible, people or situations that you know cause you a high level of distress.

7. Try to view things with a sense of perspective. How important will the particular stress situation seem in five years, or one year, or even one month?

8. Give yourself a mental pat on the back every day for some positive quality you have or express. Feel good about being you!

9. Have a sense of humor. Life can be much less stressful if you can laugh *with* others and *at* yourself.

10. Don't become rigid. Consider new ideas, meet new friends, try new experiences.

11. Have an area of interest or activity (mental or physical) outside of your work that provides pleasure and satisfaction for you.

12. Have a confidante (or group) with whom you can share your feelings, ideas and problems.

13. Don't set impossible goals or schedules for yourself—or others.

14. As best you can, keep control of your time in your own hands. Establish a reasonable schedule where others cannot constantly distract or interrupt you.

15. If you encounter a highly stressful situation, find some way to reduce the tension (walk around the block, do a relaxation technique or a breathing exercise).

16. Make sure you get enough sleep and the proper nutrition.

17. Try to view your mistakes as learning experiences rather than feeling guilty or bad about them. Forgive yourself and others.

18. Try to achieve a balance in your life between work and play; stimulation and quiet times; worrying and well-being.

19. Have a belief that there is a benevolent energy source (or higher power) that you can access.

20. And finally, remember: you may not have control over the stress situation, but you can have control over your reaction to the stress.

REPRESSION

While we don't wish this workbook to be a crash course in Psychology 101, there are some behaviors that should be explored in their relationship to overeating. Among these is repression. While its clinical meaning has a broader definition, we use this term to mean the opposite of expressing. Especially as it relates to feelings of anger, repression (that is, the holding in or attempting to ignore, deny or bury strong emotion) can result in turning to food in an attempt to relieve the feelings (to compensate). When you try to use food as a substitute for facing and expressing strong emotion, however, you find that not only are you are still stuck with the problem, you have now added the additional problem of the results of the overeating.

This isn't a suggestion to encourage temper tantrums. It is an encouragement to at least attempt to explore a concept that may help you with your overeating situation.

Men, in particular, have been conditioned to some degree by our culture to bury their emotions rather than to constructively express them or work them out. Emotions seem to be divided between "manly" and "unmanly". It's okay to get angry, but it's something else again to cry. Men are often taught that "little boys don't cry," and they then begin to identify this honest expression of feelings with something akin to horror—in their own behavior as well as that of any other "man." On the other hand, many men have never known the marvelous well-being that can come from expressions of tenderness or compassion. This doesn't mean they don't feel these things, only that they've never learned to become comfortable expressing them.

Left, then, with a festering, unexpressed and unacknowledged hurt or anger or disappointment, is it any wonder so many turn to alcohol, drugs, or food?

We encourage you to use the support group structure to communicate and to share your emotions. You may be amazed at how many others feel as you do, and who have never had the experience of talking about their strong feelings with anyone else. They may have been taught that it was unmanly or undignified to express strong emotion (which can also include the communication of love). Others have learned to express their emotion only by acts of violence such as striking out at wife or children. Anger, guilt, grief, frustration, and the like are very real emotions that we all have. Although overeating is certainly not as extreme as expressing your anger through physical violence, it is nevertheless a release for emotion that can pose some real health threats.

Many times the overwhelming anxieties you seem to be faced with are the result of not being able to express what is really bothering you. Laughter comes much easier to men than tears, and that may be unfortunate, because both represent the expression of legitimate, healthy feelings. Trying to deny to yourself that these exist only results in your burying them. They don't go away —they just sort of hang around taking little pot shots at your health and well-being. When you try to temporarily fix them with food (or drugs or alcohol), you still haven't resolved anything; you've only temporarily hidden the feelings.

Individuals who have learned to use repression as a means of trying to cope more than likely will suffer from fears and anxieties throughout their lives because they have never learned a better way to reduce their emotional tension.

Sex problems, for instance, are subjected to repression more than any other problem area. Men find it very difficult to discuss or even admit that they have sexual problems, especially in our culture. Simply because they are afraid or embarrassed to seek professional help or advice, many men suffer untold anxieties about their sexual performance, or lack of. Many men also have some totally unjustified doubts about their virility based on some rather unfortunate cultural attitudes. Most of us were taught that masturbation was abominable, or at the very least undesirable, so we can develop a whole load of guilt over what could more constructively be viewed as a natural, normal process. These unexpressed anxieties and guilt can then turn up in the form of anti-social behavior or become very real physical symptoms.

Although it sounds easier than it is to accomplish, what will work better for you is to find a way to allow and acknowledge the emotion (in an acceptable manner) and then to let it go. Many times the letting-go process is made easier by sharing it with a confidante, a support group, or turning it over to a higher power (such as your own particular version of God)—or all three. Your association with a wellness partner can be of immense help in allowing you to release, rather than to internalize your strong feelings.

In addition to communicating your feelings, it can be very beneficial to use both a focused relaxation technique and a processing technique such as we have detailed in other sections of this workbook. As you become comfortable with these new (and we hope better) ways of functioning, you may find that your desire to overeat has become greatly reduced.

PROCESSING TECHNIQUE

Sometimes when we get on edge, we tend to get a little desperate. We know we need to pull back, to release the tension, but we don't know how. At these time (which we all have), we're likely to act out of a state of disappointment, anger, or grief rather than from a state of logic and perception. This is when drugs, alcohol, food or anti-social behavior can overrule our reason.

When this happens, we need a tool—something besides the alcohol, drugs, temper outburst, or food—to put us back in balance.

One technique that can help when you experience these kinds of feelings (which by the way can also take the form of withdrawal), is what we call "processing." Processing is an easy-to-learn, easy-to-use technique that you can adapt to your specific personality needs which will allow you to release feelings that seem to overwhelm you.

When you come up against a situation that's tough to handle emotionally, there isn't a magic pill or some special incantation of words that will make it go away. However, when for whatever reason, you feel that you're emotionally under attack, processing can help put you back in control by diminishing what's eating at you.

1. You will need to find a quiet place where you can be alone for five to ten minutes. If you're at work, perhaps you will need to leave your office and take a short walk. Once you become skilled at processing, you may be able to do it in the presence of others by simply envisioning you are alone. At first, however, you will need the concentration that may be hard to achieve in the close presence of others.

2. In either a sitting or standing position, place a hand on your abdomen in the area of your diaphragm. Now breathe in and out slowly and concentrate only on how it feels to take in and blow out air. Try to think about nothing except your breathing. You can do this while walking, sitting or standing. Blow out forcefully as you exhale. Take several long, deep breaths, holding each one for a few seconds.

3. Now let out a bit of sound as you exhale. Any sound. It can be a sigh or a roar. You decide. Try to envision the muscles in the area of your diaphragm relaxing. Try to release the muscle tension from your neck and shoulders. Continue this process until you feel you are beginning to relax.

4. Once you have begun to calm down to some extent, tell yourself that it's okay to experience the strong emotion you have been feeling. Don't chastise yourself or feel guilty about your emotional reactions, and especially don't try to pretend they don't exist! Allow yourself to think about your anger or grief, but only for a minute or two.

5. Now picture all that emotion you've just been feeling flowing around in your body — circulating like your bloodstream—and then envision it flowing out through your feet into the ground. Force the emotion out slowly or send it rushing, but picture it actually leaving your body and going into the earth.

6. Silently or aloud, say "I let this feeling go" or whatever your choice of words may be. Blow out slowly. Repeat the phrase a few times.

7. Now as you envision the anger or pain flowing out, try to experience a feeling of peacefulness or well-being coming back up from the earth and going into your body. If you are outside, look at the sky or a tree. If you are inside, try looking out a window or close your eyes and see a nature scene in your mind. Create a "safe place" where you can mentally see yourself.

8. Next consider how important your anger (or whatever) will be to you in five years or even in one year. Will you even be able to remember why you were so upset? Will whatever has caused you pain even be important then? Look for a sense of perspective. Ask yourself if the unpleasant experience is important enough to jeopardize your health by internalizing it or by taking such actions as overindulging in food or drink. These behaviors will not make your pain disappear, they only provide a temporary relief that ends up causing you other problems. It doesn't work to put a bandage on a broken leg. What you really want to do is heal yourself from this temporary wound—and healing is done by letting go of the pain.

By now you should feel a little more back in control. If not, go back through the process again until you're able to better handle what was bothering you.

If necessary, call your wellness partner and share your feelings about what's bothering you. Don't repress. PROCESS OR COMMUNICATE OR BOTH!

OBSESSIVE/COMPULSIVE BEHAVIOR

One aspect of your behavior you may want to alter is compulsive behavior. Each of us has some area of compulsiveness: the difference is in degree. Some of us are compulsive about eating, others about how their socks are arranged in the bureau drawer, still others are very rigid about their schedules. There is no strict line of demarcation between what is just a mild "personality quirk" and what is dysfunctional behavior. In most cases, common sense will allow you to distinguish between the two.

The good news is that if you tend to be somewhat overly compulsive—and this compulsion manifests itself in overeating, you may be able to redirect that energy into some more positive responses. The seemingly irresistible tendency to do a specific thing (even when it is obviously not good for you) can be modified and changed to focus on a behavior that is good for you. While the ancient wisdom of moderation in all things is usually best, if your nature tends to be compulsive, you may actually have a greater chance of success than a non-compulsive person with adhering to the concepts presented in this program. It's in your nature to "stick" with something no matter what.

For instance, try trading your negative compulsion of overeating to a positive addiction of regular exercise, eating health-producing foods, getting enough rest, doing a relaxation technique. Don't, however, become obsessive and do any of these things to a degree that is harmful to you. If you have areas in your life where your extreme behavior or actions have become unmanageable enough to cause a physical or mental problem, then you should consider seeking professional counseling. Short of this, however, learning to understand why you have the compulsive need through the process of communication with your support group and/or wellness partner may be of help to you. Also using visual techniques where you see yourself being free from the compulsion may be of some help. When you are tempted to do something that is potentially harmful (i.e., excessive drinking, using drugs, food binging, etc.,) try using a relaxation technique (which can also include prayer or meditation) to reduce the urge.

No one is perfect, because perfection isn't a destination you can reach; it's a journey. Life is a trip through time where you seek to fulfill your potential, and we each do this in a different way. So you needn't necessarily view a tendency toward compulsiveness as being negative. Just do a bit of work on switching it toward a positive behavior that will help you with your wellness.

HIGHER POWER HELP

When you've got nowhere else to go for help, you may find you to need to turn to a spiritual or higher power source. You may find that turning your problem over to this source will provide you with the commitment, support and results you didn't have when you trying to do it all alone.

The reason we use the term higher power is that we each have our own idea or our own version of what this spiritual source is. You may have a very definite idea of your spiritual source and call it God. Those from other cultures call this source by different names. Some individuals are uncomfortable with the religious aspect certain words imply and are more comfortable using terms such as All That Is, total consciousness, nature, energy, or simply joy. The word you use is not what is important. What is important is that you believe that you can access some higher aspect of power within yourself or a source that you believe resides outside of you. This is not an attempt to get you involved in religion; it's a hint to you to use some form of spirituality to make the challenge you're faced with here a little easier.

This kind of philosophy works well with the behavior modifications we have suggested because you can use a spiritual meditation or prayer form of focused relaxation, and you can also use spiritual affirmations. Ask your higher power source for help to:

- Release negative feelings about yourself and others

- Forgive and be forgiven as a method of clearing guilt and anger

- Heal your body

- Allow you to change attitudes about your body and your weight

- Give you strength and commitment

- Receive guidance in properly nourishing your body

For many, the idea that they can turn control of their eating over to a higher source is the difference between success and failure with a weight-loss plan. They are able to develop the belief —which then becomes reality—that they are both deserving and capable of having a trim, healthy body.

As a suggestion, you could use some of the following affirmations.

I, _____ , turn my body over to (your higher power source) and ask for guidance with my wellness program.

Because I, _____ , have the guidance of (my higher power source) I am able to choose food that makes me healthy.

I, _____ , turn my eating problems over to (higher power source) and know that with this help I will achieve my wellness goals.

Each of you will have his own belief and appropriate words regarding your source of spiritual help. Try using this source to give thanks, to forgive and to be forgiven, and to ask for help.

V

MONITORING

MONITORING

Now that you have better knowledge of all the aspects involved in your BALANCE wellness program, you are ready to begin to actively accomplish your weight-loss goal.

A daily activity log sheet (which includes a food diary) has been provided in this section. You need to fill out one of these sheets each day. (Please photocopy extra sheets as needed.) It includes:

1. A section for what you plan to eat as well as what you actually eat during the day.

2. A place to list weight and measurements.

3. A check-off listing for worksheet activities that you have completed each day, plus your relaxation technique and eating affirmations.

4. A check-off listing for your physical exercises.

It is important that you use this log on a daily basis. It will help you stick to your schedule and keep you actively reminded of what you are trying to accomplish.

On a separate worksheet there is also a chart on which you can keep a progressive record of your weight loss.

Please make additional copies of these two sheets as they are needed.

WHY A FOOD DIARY?

A food diary may seem to be a nuisance, but the reality is that unless you record every mouthful, you're not going to have an accurate picture of what you are consuming. Acquiring the habit of writing down what you eat will make you more aware of how much and what kinds of food you are eating. So, even though it does seem like a nuisance, it is an important part of your wellness program and does serve a two-fold purpose.

1. It helps you monitor what you eat: the quantities, the calories or the exchanges within the limits you set for yourself.

2. The process of writing it down creates an awareness of and allows control over the nutritional aspect of your life.

At some future point in time, it may not be necessary for you to keep a written tally of everything you eat, but you will still be doing it as a mental process. In other words, you will be so used to knowing calories or exchange values, as well as portions, that you will mentally be able to keep a record of what and how much you eat every day.

The log sheet contains both a "food forecast" and an "actual food eaten" section. The forecast column will provide a daily road map for you, and will also aid you in your shopping. You must fill out both the forecast and the actual. Don't worry if from time to time your actual deviates from your forecast. You are bound to encounter situations where you will need to make some adjustments. And remember, you are removing the unnecessary fats and sugars, so focus on not only what you are eating, but how it is prepared. See "Eating Out" and "Cooking" sections for more detail.

Concentrate on eating nutritionally. Make sure you include all the required food groups each day. If you overeat one day, cut back for a couple of days. Even though you are keeping track of your calories or exchanges on a daily basis, the total at the end of the week is what is most important. That doesn't mean you should starve one day and gorge the next. That kind of eating will not bring you wellness.

For many individuals, it works best to do your forecast section a week at a time, and to do the actual section after each meal. By having a forecast done ahead of time, you will be able to make sure you have the right foods on hand to eat. If you're tired or stressed out, it's difficult to also have to do meal planning. If you have already decided what to have for dinner, and your food is in the cupboard or refrigerator, you will have a better chance of sticking with your food plan. If you don't know what you're going to eat, you will probably eat something you shouldn't.

DAILY ACTIVITY LOG
(please photocopy extra sheets)

DATE

WATER (circle # of glasses) A.M. 1 2 3 4 5 P.M. 1 2 3 4 5

FOOD FORECAST	**CALORIES OR EXCHANGES**
Breakfast	
Lunch	
Dinner	
Snack(s)	
Total	

FOOD DIARY	
Breakfast	
Lunch	
Dinner	
Snack(s)	
Total	

FOOD GROUPS (check if included)

Protein _____ Vegetables _____ Fruits _____ Starches _____ Dairy _____

WEIGHT (daily or weekly, as appropriate) _____

MEASUREMENTS (weekly or monthly) Chest _____ Waist _____ Hips _____

WORKSHEET ACTIVITIES (specify which ones) _____

FOCUSED RELAXATION TECHNIQUE (check off if done) _____

EATING AFFIRMATION (check off if done) _____

EXERCISE (check if done)	**ELAPSED TIME**
Aerobic	
Strengthening	
Stretching	

DAILY ACTIVITY LOG
(please photocopy extra sheets)

DATE

WATER (circle # of glasses) A.M. 1 2 3 4 5 P.M. 1 2 3 4 5

FOOD FORECAST   **CALORIES OR EXCHANGES**

Breakfast _____   _____

Lunch _____   _____

Dinner _____   _____

Snack(s) _____   _____

Total   _____

FOOD DIARY

Breakfast _____   _____

Lunch _____   _____

Dinner _____   _____

Snack(s) _____   _____

Total   _____

FOOD GROUPS (check if included)

Protein _____ Vegetables _____ Fruits _____ Starches _____ Dairy _____

WEIGHT (daily or weekly, as appropriate) _____

MEASUREMENTS (weekly or monthly) Chest _____ Waist _____ Hips _____

WORKSHEET ACTIVITIES (specify which ones) _____

FOCUSED RELAXATION TECHNIQUE (check off if done) _____

EATING AFFIRMATION (check off if done) _____

EXERCISE (check if done)   **ELAPSED TIME**

Aerobic _____   _____

Strengthening _____   _____

Stretching _____   _____

DAILY ACTIVITY LOG
(please photocopy extra sheets)

DATE _____

WATER (circle # of glasses) A.M. 1 2 3 4 5 P.M. 1 2 3 4 5

FOOD FORECAST   **CALORIES OR EXCHANGES**

Breakfast _____   _____

Lunch _____   _____

Dinner _____   _____

Snack(s) _____   _____

                                    Total   _____

FOOD DIARY

Breakfast _____   _____

Lunch _____   _____

Dinner _____   _____

Snack(s) _____   _____

                                    Total   _____

FOOD GROUPS (check if included)

Protein _____   Vegetables _____   Fruits _____   Starches _____   Dairy _____

WEIGHT (daily or weekly, as appropriate) _____

MEASUREMENTS (weekly or monthly) Chest _____ Waist _____ Hips _____

WORKSHEET ACTIVITIES (specify which ones) _____

FOCUSED RELAXATION TECHNIQUE (check off if done) _____

EATING AFFIRMATION (check off if done) _____

EXERCISE (check if done)   **ELAPSED TIME**

Aerobic _____   _____

Strengthening _____   _____

Stretching _____   _____

DAILY ACTIVITY LOG
(please photocopy extra sheets)

DATE

WATER (circle # of glasses) A.M. 1 2 3 4 5 P.M. 1 2 3 4 5

FOOD FORECAST	**CALORIES OR EXCHANGES**
Breakfast	
Lunch	
Dinner	
Snack(s)	
Total	

FOOD DIARY	
Breakfast	
Lunch	
Dinner	
Snack(s)	
Total	

FOOD GROUPS (check if included)

Protein _____   Vegetables _____   Fruits _____   Starches _____   Dairy _____

WEIGHT (daily or weekly, as appropriate) _____

MEASUREMENTS (weekly or monthly) Chest _____   Waist _____   Hips _____

WORKSHEET ACTIVITIES (specify which ones) _____

FOCUSED RELAXATION TECHNIQUE (check off if done) _____

EATING AFFIRMATION (check off if done) _____

EXERCISE (check if done)	**ELAPSED TIME**
Aerobic	
Strengthening	
Stretching	

DAILY ACTIVITY LOG
(please photocopy extra sheets)

DATE

WATER (circle # of glasses) A.M. 1 2 3 4 5 P.M. 1 2 3 4 5

FOOD FORECAST   **CALORIES OR EXCHANGES**

Breakfast _____   _____

Lunch _____   _____

Dinner _____   _____

Snack(s) _____   _____

                              Total   _____

FOOD DIARY

Breakfast _____   _____

Lunch _____   _____

Dinner _____   _____

Snack(s) _____   _____

                              Total   _____

FOOD GROUPS (check if included)

Protein _____   Vegetables _____   Fruits _____   Starches _____   Dairy _____

WEIGHT (daily or weekly, as appropriate)_____

MEASUREMENTS (weekly or monthly) Chest _____ Waist _____ Hips _____

WORKSHEET ACTIVITIES (specify which ones) _____

FOCUSED RELAXATION TECHNIQUE (check off if done) _____

EATING AFFIRMATION (check off if done) _____

EXERCISE (check if done)   **ELAPSED TIME**

Aerobic   _____   _____

Strengthening   _____   _____

Stretching   _____   _____

DAILY ACTIVITY LOG
(please photocopy extra sheets)

DATE

WATER (circle # of glasses) A.M. 1 2 3 4 5   P.M. 1 2 3 4 5

FOOD FORECAST	**CALORIES OR EXCHANGES**
Breakfast	
Lunch	
Dinner	
Snack(s)	
Total	

FOOD DIARY	
Breakfast	
Lunch	
Dinner	
Snack(s)	
Total	

FOOD GROUPS (check if included)

Protein _____ Vegetables _____ Fruits _____ Starches _____ Dairy _____

WEIGHT (daily or weekly, as appropriate)_____

MEASUREMENTS (weekly or monthly) Chest _____ Waist _____ Hips _____

WORKSHEET ACTIVITIES (specify which ones) _____

FOCUSED RELAXATION TECHNIQUE (check off if done) _____

EATING AFFIRMATION (check off if done) _____

EXERCISE (check if done)	**ELAPSED TIME**
Aerobic	
Strengthening	
Stretching	

DAILY ACTIVITY LOG
(please photocopy extra sheets)

DATE

WATER (circle # of glasses) A.M. 1 2 3 4 5 P.M. 1 2 3 4 5

FOOD FORECAST   **CALORIES OR EXCHANGES**

Breakfast _____   _____

Lunch _____   _____

Dinner _____   _____

Snack(s) _____   _____

                                   Total   _____

FOOD DIARY

Breakfast _____   _____

Lunch _____   _____

Dinner _____   _____

Snack(s) _____   _____

                                   Total   _____

FOOD GROUPS (check if included)

Protein _____   Vegetables _____   Fruits _____   Starches _____   Dairy _____

WEIGHT (daily or weekly, as appropriate) _____

MEASUREMENTS (weekly or monthly) Chest _____ Waist _____ Hips _____

WORKSHEET ACTIVITIES (specify which ones) _____

FOCUSED RELAXATION TECHNIQUE (check off if done) _____

EATING AFFIRMATION (check off if done) _____

EXERCISE (check if done)   **ELAPSED TIME**

Aerobic _____   _____

Strengthening _____   _____

Stretching _____   _____

WEIGHING AND MEASURING YOURSELF AND WEIGHT PLATEAUS

The frequency with which you weigh is a very individual matter. Some programs require that you weigh every day; some recommend weighing only once a week. If you do weigh yourself daily, be sure you do it at the same time each day wearing clothing of approximately the same weight each time. Your weight can fluctuate as much as four pounds from morning till evening, and depending upon how much fluid you are retaining, can also fluctuate from day to day. For this reason, we recommend that if you are going to be on a long-term weight loss program, you will usually find it works better for you if you weigh weekly. However, you will want to decide whether you should weigh daily, weekly, or monthly.

The chart on the following page should be used to keep track of your progress. Note that in addition to your weight (which you record weekly), you will need to also list your measurements on a weekly or monthly basis. There will be times when, according to your scales, your weight reaches a plateau for a period of time. This is a normal phenomenon and should not be considered failure on your part to lose weight as long as you are following your food plan. If you check your measurements during this weight plateau you will usually find that you have continued to lose inches and that your clothes are looser. Plateaus can be encountered every three to four weeks, so don't get discouraged. During the following week or two you will probably see a fairly encouraging drop in your weight.

One thing that can sometimes be at the root of your plateau situation is not drinking enough water. If you're not drinking 8 to 10 glasses of water a day, you will slow the weight process down or even retain fluid. If this is your case, get back on your water regimen! (See section on water for details.)

While your bathroom scales may tell you how much you weigh, they cannot tell you how that weight is distributed into fat, muscle and water. A better indicator of your overall fitness level is your body fat ratio. For men, a desirable body fat level should be under 18%.

The healthy body is approximately 50% water (by weight), but when you lose weight too rapidly, what you lose is not fat, but water; you upset this healthy water balance and pull water from your lean muscle and other vital body tissues. This kind of weight loss is not fat loss, and it quickly replaces itself as you return to normal eating. When losing weight, you want to keep from losing lean tissue and skeletal muscle. This is why when you lose too quickly you get sagging skin. Your "frame" shrinks, seeming to leave you with too much skin. How your total weight breaks down by percentage is a more accurate indicator of your desired weight level and physical condition than just knowing your total weight. After all, 50 pounds of muscle is certainly more attractive than 50 pounds of fat, but they both weigh the same an your bathroom scale. The best way to determine your body fat ratio is by hydrostatic (or underwater) weighing, although caliper measurement can also give a fairly accurate reading.

WEEKLY WEIGHT-LOSS AND MEASUREMENT CHART

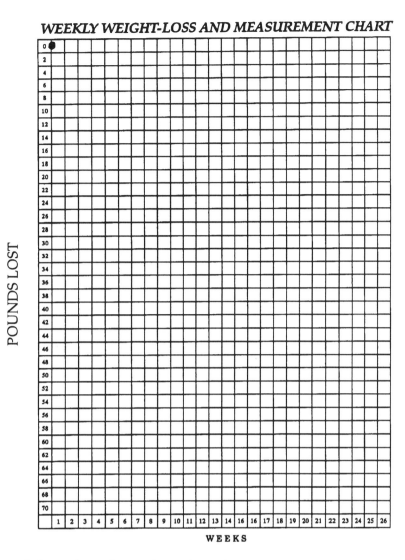

Starting at top left, make a dot each week at the appropriate intersection of pounds lost and the number of weeks you have been on your program. The first dot has been made for you at 0. At the end of week one, weigh yourself and record your loss by putting a dot above week one opposite the appropriate amount of weight loss. Connect your dots with a line from week to week to show your weight loss.

RECORD WEEKLY MEASUREMENTS BELOW (INCHES)

MEASUREMENT

CHEST	___	___	___	___	___	___	___	___	___	___
WAIST	___	___	___	___	___	___	___	___	___	___
HIPS	___	___	___	___	___	___	___	___	___	___
WEEK #	1	2	3	4	5	6	7	8	9	10

SEMI-FAST

When you're stuck at a weight plateau or you've overindulged and need to make up for it, a one-day semi-fast may be your answer. Remember, this is only for one day; don't continue it for several days because it doesn't contain the nutritional requirements your body needs.

1. Six apples spread throughout the day. If you can't handle any more sweet taste by the end of the day, substitute a tomato or a glass of tomato juice or vegetable juice for one of the apples.

2. An all-vegetable day which can include any veggie, including one baked potato, (not a yam or sweet potato), or any kind of squash. Do not eat any beans (except green), corn, or peas. Use lemon or vinegar on salad. Use any herb or spice. Veggies can be raw or cooked (or both).

3. A vegetable and fruit day which includes as much as you want of any vegetable (except those restricted above) or fruit. As a suggestion, you might want to have fruit for breakfast, a vegetable salad plus fruit for lunch, and a baked potato plus a fruit dessert for dinner.

WHAT IF I HAVE A LAPSE?

An important fact to realize about yourself and everyone else is that perfection is not a destination—it's a journey. That's what living is all about: learning, experiencing, creating and conquering challenges. Weight-loss objectives are in some respects no different than other objectives you set for yourself.

You are now headed down the road of health and wellness. This doesn't mean that if you temporarily wander off the path that you're not still headed for your destination. Sometimes we set ourselves up for feelings of failure because we choose to challenge ourselves in unrealistic ways. We believe that if we deviate from our "perfect" plan, then we should consider ourselves failures. Don't set yourself up with this kind of thinking. If you view your wellness plan as an either/or situation or as a win/lose situation, you're already programming yourself for failure.

Wellness is an ongoing process. It's a journey. On some days, for whatever reason (your own or someone else's), you're going to deviate from your plan. This is not failure, nor is it an excuse to bag the whole thing. You can either view obstacles you encounter in your life and in this program as problems or as opportunities. The glass can be either half empty or half full.

If you do go off the program for a few days, a few weeks, or even a few months, all you need to do is make a decision to take up where you left off, then do it! Take it one day at a time. The side excursion may have taught you something about yourself that will be of help at a later date.

On the other hand, don't abuse this kind of philosophy and use it as a excuse for overeating or for eating the wrong foods. That's counterproductive to what *you* have chosen to accomplish. Use the experience for positive reinforcement. Forgive yourself, view it as an opportunity to learn, let go of any negative feelings about it—and get on with your program and with your life!

Go back and review or redo any activity sheets that will put you back on track. Call your wellness partner. Review your commitment. Remember: one day at a time. Yesterday is already gone. Concentrate on today.

WHY I HAD A LAPSE

1. Why do I think I went off my program?

2. Is there something I've learned about myself or others that can help me avoid this in the future?

3. What could I have done instead of going off my program?

4. If I'm tempted to go off again, what can I do to help reinforce my commitment to stick with it?

REWARD YOURSELF ACTIVITY

1. If there were no limitations on your time and you had a day when you didn't have to do anything except just exactly what *you* wanted to do, what would it be:

2. Consider setting some interim goals for your weight loss program such as 10 pounds (or whatever you decide is a reasonable benchmark.) When you achieve one of these goals, reward yourself by allowing yourself to do what you have listed in #1 above (as far as possible).

3. What one small thing (related to time or money) could you do for yourself that would give you a sense of gratification (i.e., professional shave, massage, haircut, manicure, new tie, shoe shine, new book, a soak in the hot tub, a movie, fishing, etc.)?

4. Allow yourself to do the activity in #3 above when you need a reward or when you're feeling like you need some positive reinforcement.

VI

PHYSICAL FITNESS

PHYSICAL FITNESS

We cannot stress too strongly that exercise is an absolutely essential part of your wellness program. Without it, your basal metabolism rate will drop, and you will not be able to keep off the weight you have worked so hard to lose. It's not easy to find time or to make the commitment, but you must find a way to fit exercise into your daily schedule. Remember, you also need your doctor's permission before you begin so that you can assure you aren't doing or causing any damage.

Exercise is necessary not only to help your body burn stored fat, it is also necessary for good health. You don't need a strenuous or lengthy regimen in order to help you burn fat or to achieve fitness. In fact, too much anaerobic exercise (which means without air such as strenuous calisthenics, heavy weight lifting, etc.) will only burn your necessary supply of stored glucose rather than your supply of stored fat.

Complete physical fitness includes endurance, strength, and flexibility. Your exercise program should include activities that will contribute to all three aspects of fitness.

An aerobic exercise (i.e., continuous, rhythmic, air-using) is the most beneficial for weight loss. This includes continuous activity such as walking, running, bicycling, and swimming. For the most part, the exercise received in tennis and similar sports does not provide enough continuous motion to be classified as aerobic. While a certain amount of the proper kind of anaerobic exercise is desirable for strength and toning, you must have the beneficial heart and lung activity that can only come from an exercise that gets and keep your pulse rate up to a specific target zone. You need a minimum of at least 20 continuous minutes per day at this rate (not counting warm-up and cool-down periods of from 5 to 10 minutes each) to achieve the kind of aerobic benefit you need.

The ideal fat-burning state is when the heart rate (pulse) is at between 60% and 85% of the maximum heart rate for your age. The best formula to use to determine this is as follows. First you must know your resting heart rate which is your pulse rate when you first awake (before getting out of bed). Measure your pulse for 15 seconds and then multiply by 4. Then continue with the formula.

1. 220 minus your age equals maximum heart rate

2. Maximum heart rate minus resting pulse rate

3. Multiply this figure by both 60% and by 85% to give you the low and high range of your target zone.

4. Add back your resting heart rate.

You can use a shortened version of this formula by subtracting your age from 220. Multiply that figure by 60% to get your minimum target heart rate an 85% to get your maximum target heart rate. (This shortened formula is not as accurate, however, as when you also include your resting heart rate as shown in the example below.)

E.G.   220

    <u>-48</u> (your age)

    172 (maximum heart rate)

    <u>-60</u> (resting pulse rate)

    112

    <u>x60%</u> (for minimum workout)

     67

    <u>+48</u> (age)

    115 (minimum target zone)

• •

    112

    <u>x85%</u> (maximum workout)

     95

    <u>+48</u> (age)

    143 (maximum target zone)

You will want to check your resting pulse rate periodically because as you lose weight and get in better physical condition, your pulse rate will tend to drop. Especially when you are first starting an exercise program, it isn't advisable to go as high as 85%. That's the highest it should ever be. Past that rate and you are endangering your health. A sustained rate of 70% will actually produce more fat burning than the higher rate.

You should plan for at least five exercise sessions per week as a minimum. While on a weight-reduction program, it is best if you do some kind of sustained activity for at least 30 minutes on a daily basis. (Some experts recommend taking off one day a week to allow your body to rest and restore.)

When you are first beginning an exercise program, start at 50% to 60% of your target heart rate, then gradually increase to 70% as you get in better condition. Remember, you can't do it overnight! The true test of your fitness level is your recovery rate, that is, how quickly you can return to a normal pulse rate after sustained activity.

You will burn approximately 8 calories per minute when you reach your target rate (70%). Your body will burn another 50 or so calories returning to your normal pulse rate. You will be strengthening your most important muscle—your heart.

Increasing muscle strength can be done with a good routine of light calisthenics or light (hand-held) weights. There are several excellent books and video tapes on the market that can be of help in developing your own regimen. Again, the workout need not be overly strenuous or lengthy. It is more important that you do it on a regular basis. Good results can be expected from a moderate workout 3 or 4 times a week.

One note of caution. Incorrectly done, these kinds of exercises can cause damage. Until you are confident that you are doing them correctly, either observe yourself in a full-length mirror or have someone watch you. You need to do anaerobic exercise properly in order to avoid injury. Flexibility can be accomplished by doing proper stretching before and after both aerobic and anaerobic activity.

Listed below is a chart of average calorie usage in various aerobic activities based on a half hour of participation by a 160 pound man.

ACTIVITY	CALORIE LOSS
Aerobic dance	300
Bicycling (moderately)	130
Bicycling (vigorously)	300
Climbing stairs	175
Jogging	275
Running	450
Swimming (vigorously)	350
Walking (moderately)	105
Walking (vigorously)	170

One approach to exercise you may want to use in developing your wellness program is one of trading compulsions. Many of us (especially the type A personalities) tend to be somewhat compulsive. This is not necessarily a disadvantage in a weight-loss program, because with a "stick-to-it" mind set approach, you can train yourself to trade your compulsive overeating for the "positive addiction" of exercise. This is not an invitation to become a marathon runner or to put your exercise level totally out of proportion so that you subject yourself to either short-term or long-term injury. It is an opportunity, however, for you to use energy in a more healthy manner.

You do need to be wary of the kind of thinking that goes "if a little bit is good, then a lot must be better." As with most things in life, exercise should be done with some degree of moderation. Done to excess, it can cause health problems rather than providing the benefits you are seeking.

Symptoms such as chest pain, abnormal heart rhythm, headaches, urinary bleeding, heartburn, nausea, vomiting and diarrhea can all result from exercise abuse. Heavy exercisers can put themselves at risk of osteoporosis (yes, men as well as women), mood disorders such as depression, and eating disorders such as anorexia or bulimia. In addition, you run the very real risk of sustaining injuries such as muscle and tendon damage, sprains, plus bone and joint problems.

Exercising in order to achieve strength, flexibility and endurance does not mean you are in a contest. Leave the "jock mentality" for others. A well-balanced, reasonable, regular regimen will prove more beneficial than exercising to excess. Running, for example, isn't for everyone. Those who have certain types of structural conditions are susceptible to foot and knee problems that can become so aggravated by running as to prohibit them from engaging in almost any kind of exercise regimen. Aerobic-level walking, for instance, can provide as much benefit as running, while greatly reducing your chances for injury.

The belief of "no pain, no gain" has been proven to be a myth. If your body is experiencing pain, it has been over stressed and you are more likely to experience injury. If you push yourself too hard, you may have to give up exercising while you recover, and that's not going to help you lose weight.

Choose a type of exercise that you enjoy doing or you won't stick with it long. You may need the extra incentive of an exercise partner who encourages you to stick with your program. For some, the regimen provided by signing up for a class or joining a fitness facility provides incentive.

If possible, try to do some portion of your exercise program out of doors and use this time to also relax your mind. A park or a setting where there is pleasant scenery can provide a peaceful environment that can encourage you to combine your physical exercise with mental relaxation. Perhaps your exercise time can be your special time alone when you process the day's frustrations or experiences by exchanging them for a feeling of tranquillity and well-being.

WALKING

After a decade of fascination with jogging and running, walking has now become the exercise of choice for many. If you have not engaged in any form of regular aerobic exercise for a while, we recommend that you start off your physical fitness program with walking. As you get in better physical condition, running is certainly an option you can consider, but it is important that you don't try to overdo the process of getting in shape by overextending your capacity. While running is still a popular form of exercise, it has also produced such an abundance of injuries that sports medicine clinics now abound. You can get just as much benefit from walking as you can from running if you maintain a brisk pace. Walking at 3.5 to 4 miles per hour burns nearly as many calories as running at a moderate pace. It just takes longer to walk your two or three (or more) miles than it does to run. Walking is an inexpensive, healthy and pleasant form of needed daily exercise.

As you begin your involvement with the physical fitness portion of the BALANCE program, we recommend you try to walk a minimum of five days per week. Seven is even better. Pick a route that is pleasant and let the view or scenery help your mind relax while your body is working. You may want to vary your route so it doesn't become monotonous. It may help you maintain your dedication if you have a walking partner who can help provide you with motivation. Establish a regular time for your walk and stick with it. It's tougher on stormy days, but it is important that you make and keep your commitment.

You should be sure to include a warm-up and some stretches that will help your muscles become more flexible. Remember that physical fitness includes flexibility as well as strength and endurance. First, walk for a few minutes at your normal pace, then work up to a more brisk rate. This warm-up walk should be from 5 to 10 minutes. After you have warmed up your muscles, you will need to stretch the hamstrings, calves, Achilles tendons, as well as your arms and torso. NEVER STRETCH COLD MUSCLES. ALWAYS WARM UP FIRST.

STRETCHING EXERCISES:

1. Hamstring Stretch

With feet about six inches apart and knees straight (not locked), bend forward slowly and reach for the ground. Stretch as far as you can with arms dangling. Breathe deeply and don't bounce. Hold your stretch for about 20 seconds, then come up slowly. Repeat this several times trying to get closer to the ground each time.

2. Calf and Achilles Tendon Stretch

Stand back at arm's length from a wall or tree with both hands on the wall (or tree). Move your right foot back one step, then keeping your heels on the ground, lean forward with your back straight until you can feel you are stretching the right calf muscle. Breathe deeply and hold this position for about 20 seconds, then relax and repeat with the left foot.

3. Arm and torso stretch

With feet about shoulder distance apart, bend your right arm and place it on the back of your neck. Now take a hold of your right elbow with your left hand and slowly pull it toward your ear until you feel a gentle stretch. Breathe deeply and hold the stretch for about 20 seconds. Repeat with the left arm.

Now that you have warmed up and stretched, you are ready for your walk. It is important that you have shoes that fit comfortably and that are flexible. There are some excellent athletic shoes made specifically for walking, and there are also athletic shoes that are multi-purpose. Wear clothing that is loose and comfortable. Layered clothing works well because you can shed the outer layer as you get warmed up.

After your warm-up period, start walking briskly and continue for thirty minutes. If you feel you are getting too tired, slow down a bit until you catch your breath, but try to do a minimum of thirty minutes. After you get in better shape you can add additional time onto your schedule.

At the end of your walk you should stretch again for a few minutes. This will keep your muscles from getting sore and will help you maintain flexibility. Use the same stretch exercises you did at the beginning of your walk.

Remember that the key to physical fitness is regularity. For anyone on weight-loss program, it's a crucial part of the process. Without it you are subjecting yourself to a lowered metabolic rate which will more than likely result in your gaining back the weight you have worked so hard to lose. After you have reached your weight-loss objective, you can drop back to three or four days per week, but during the time when you are trying to lose weight, your body will accomplish this much more efficiently if you exercise daily. Regular exercise is a key factor in your long-term wellness.

As you walk, remain erect; don't bend forward. Let your arms swing naturally. Try to hold in stomach muscles and don't round your shoulders. If you feel you are in good condition, you may want to add one-pound wrist weights and swing your arms vigorously. Without arm pumping action, the weights don't provide much benefit.

If you are just beginning an exercise program, a rate of three miles per hour for 30 minutes is about right. (That's approximately a mile and a half.) As you become more fit, try for 45 minutes at 3.5 miles per hour, and then try to increase to one hour at a brisk 4 to 4.5 miles per hour (four to four and one-half miles).

Your cardiovascular system will get the most benefit if you are within your target heart rate (60% to 85% of your maximum heart rate).

WALKING SPEED CONVERSION TABLE

MINUTES PER MILE	MILES PER HOUR
30	2.0
24	2.5
20	3.0
17	3.5
15	4.0
13	4.5
12	5.0
11	5.5
10	6.0

There are many options for walkers:

RACE WALKING

Race walking is one form of walking that is gaining in popularity. It differs from regular walking where you take parallel steps. In race walking you put one foot in front of the other in an almost straight line and you swing your hips forward creating a rolling gait. You should pump each arm forward while swiveling the opposite hip outward. Take long strides and pump your arms vigorously to counteract your hip motion. It takes some practice, but advocates swear by it.

POLE WALKING

Pole walking is like cross country skiing without the skis. You use a rubber tipped walking stick sold in sporting goods stores. This form of walking helps exercise the upper body as well as the legs.

STRIDING

This is a sort of enlarged form of walking where you exaggerate your stride length, swing your arms freely, and try for a faster pace. You can also incorporate vigorous pumping of bent elbows (90 degree angle) into striding, similar to the arm form used in race walking.

HILL WALKING

Combine hills with flat terrain walking for aesthetic variety as well as an increase in the intensity of exercise. Lean a bit forward going up hill and take shortened steps on the way down to reduce joint stress.

RETRO WALKING

Walking backwards works different muscle groups than ordinary forward walking. Be sure to choose a smooth surface away from traffic. A partner to guide you is helpful. Use this for variety as a part of a total walking program.

VII

STABILIZATION
AND
MAINTENANCE

STABILIZATION

Now that you have reached your weight-loss goal, you will want to continue to be a person without a weight problem. You will want to incorporate the new habits and knowledge about yourself and food into a permanent lifestyle. By now you realize that being healthy is what weight loss is all about, and that you can choose to STAY IN BALANCE!

First, (and this is extremely important), you will need to *gradually* readjust your eating. It will take your body a minimum of from three to four weeks to make the chemical adjustments necessary to allow you to go on your maintenance program. If you don't go through this readjustment period using moderation in your eating, you may quickly replace old habits that you have worked so hard to retrain and find that you are regaining the weight you worked so hard to lose. Keeping excess weight off is not an easy task. It requires commitment and diligence.

In order to stabilize your system, you should now gradually begin adding additional quantities of food. It is important to remember:

1. To continue to drink a minimum of 8 glasses of water daily.

2. The key to appetite control is keeping your blood sugar level stabilized.

3. You must continue with your daily exercise program. (When you go on to the maintenance portion of your program you should be able to reduce this to three or four times a week if you wish.)

4. You still need to eliminate excess fat as well as refined sugar and flour.

During week one, add an additional daily fruit. Increase your starch allowance during week two to 4 slices or cups (or 4 servings per day). Add an additional one-cup dairy serving during week three. You can also incorporate these foods groups in a reversed order, if you choose. That is, you can increase your starch during week one, your dairy choice during week two, and your fruit during week three. Just don't add all three increases at one time and overload your "adjustment" mechanisms.

Make sure you monitor your weight during this period. If you increase your quantity too abruptly, you are going to gain weight. This gradual approach to weight stabilization is important because during this period your system will be undergoing changes. Don't overload or you will undo a lot of dedication and effort that has resulted in achieving your weight-loss goals.

At the end of this three-week period, you can begin a more relaxed maintenance program such as the one suggested on the following pages.

Congratulations on reaching your desired weight level. This is a marvelous achievement which you richly deserve!

MAINTENANCE

Congratulations! You have achieved a goal that represents extraordinary dedication and commitment. You deserve the highest praise for what you have accomplished.

You have developed new knowledge about food and about yourself, and you have adopted a new way of eating that helps you look and feel wonderful. So where do you go from here?

For many, reaching their weight-loss goal is not the hardest part of wellness; maintaining their weight loss is the stickler. There are several reasons for this. For one, when you have a particular weight-loss amount in mind, it is usually also connected to a time span. That is, you know you have to really watch what you eat, but if you do, you will ultimately get where you are headed. You can see the light at the end of the tunnel, as it were. However, once you get to where you were headed, the maintenance seems to loom ahead of you forever. There doesn't appear to be a light at the end of the tunnel; the journey seems unending. And this is where many of us tend to have problems. It's easy to develop an attitude of just one more won't hurt, or just a couple of days of eating whatever I want won't matter. The problem is that this kind of thinking can add up to lots of pounds.

Part of what you have accomplished with your food plan is retraining your appetite. However, it doesn't take much for it to slip back to its old ways. So even though you can now relax a bit, eat a bit more, and add foods that you didn't eat while on your weight-loss plan, you don't want to go back to eating the way you did when you had a weight problem. Here are some suggestions that will help you to continue to be a person without a weight problem.

1. Try to take your life one day at a time. Try not to view an unending tunnel in front of you where you feel you can never eat the things you know you shouldn't eat.

2. Learn where and when you can make trade-offs. If you overeat on the weekend, for instance, cut back during the week.

3. Rather than feeling like you have failed when you gain a few pounds, learn to allow periodic small weight fluctuations. Be sure to set a limit, though (say five pounds) and then go back on your program for a few days until you reach your desired weight.

4. Learn to listen and to trust your body. It knows when it is full; it knows what nutrients you need if you stop and listen. Don't eat when you're not really hungry, and stop eating *before* you are completely full.

5. Make sure you continue to drink 8 to 10 glasses of water. Believe it or not, this one simple step is, for many, the key to weight maintenance.

6. Continue to exercise at least 30 minutes three times per week.

7. Take some quality time for yourself every day. Do some type of focused relaxation technique daily. Use this time to process your stress rather than using food.

8. Continue to "cook light." By now you know this doesn't mean having to give up delicious meals. Use low-calorie equivalents to offset cravings for high-calorie foods.

9. Continue to weigh yourself regularly. For some, weighing monthly works best, for others, weighing weekly is more effective.

10. Continue to believe that you are entitled and deserving of wellness.

Try not to become obsessed with your weight and with your eating. That kind of behavior puts you under unnecessary stress and can lead to health problems. You have proven that **you** are in control of your behavior and your life. Now try to relax and enjoy it. Wellness is an on-going process that must include feelings of satisfaction rather than feelings of continued deprivation. This is why food education and an exercise program you can live with are critical. If you try to create goals and objectives that are not realistic, if you set yourself up with too many "forever forbiddens" or an overly excessive fitness regimen, you are also setting yourself up for some problems. You need realistic, reasonable eating and exercise goals—food that you like and exercise that you enjoy.

Remember that you are seeking balance and harmony in your life, not a roller coaster ride between eating and starving.

EATING NUTRITIONALLY

While there are several sources that give information on nutritional requirements, we have listed here the U.S. government's Recommended Dietary Allowance (RDA) as well as recommendations from the American Heart Association (related to cholesterol levels).

From a health-maintenance standpoint, no more than 30% (preferably less) of your daily food intake should be fat (which includes saturated animal fats as well as polyunsaturated vegetable sources). On a weight-loss program, it is recommended that you consume no more than 10 to 20% fat. The adult male needs only 56 grams of protein daily (from meat as well as other food sources). The remainder of your diet should be made up of carbohydrates, preferably complex or unrefined. There is controversy over whether or not an adult actually needs or benefits from dairy products, but if you do include these in your meals or snacks, try to use non-fat choices. Maintenance calories for a man average 2,500 calories per day, although this may vary depending upon height, age, and activity level.

In very general terms, dietary maintenance (not weight-loss) requirements should include the following.

RDA GUIDELINES:

Category of Food	Portion per Day
Bread, cereal, pasta, rice	6 to 11 servings
Vegetables	3 to 5 servings
Fruit	2 to 4 servings
Protein (meat, poultry, fish, eggs, dried beans/peas)	2 to 3 servings
Dairy (milk, yogurt, cheese)	2 to 3 servings
Fats, oil, and sweets	Use sparingly

AMERICAN HEART ASSOCIATION GUIDELINES

To control the amount and kind of fat you eat:

• Limit your intake of meat, seafood and poultry to no more than 6 ounces per day.

• Use chicken or turkey (without skin) or fish in most of your main meals.

• Choose lean cuts of meat, trim all the fat you can see, and throw away the fat that cooks out of the meat.

• Substitute meatless or "low-meat" main dishes for regular entrees.

• Use no more than a total of 5-8 teaspoons of fats and oils per day for cooking, baking and salads.

To control your intake of cholesterol-rich foods:

• Use no more than four egg yolks a week, including those used in cooking.

• Limit your use of shrimp, lobster and organ meat.

GET MORE BOOKS FROM R & E AND SAVE!

TITLES	ORDER #	PRICE
Balance: The Wellness and Weight-Control Primer for Men *Motivational techninques and strategies for health*	065-X	$11.95
The First Law Enforcement Cookbook *Have Badge Will Cook! Great Recipes For Anyone*	063-3	$7.95
All American Cooking *Savory Recipes From Savvy Cooks Across America*	902-4	$7.95
The Lowfat Mexican Cookbook *True Mexican Taste Without The Waist*	896-6	$6.95
Practical Fat-Free Living *A Guide To Simple Life-Long, Life-Style Changes*		
The Recreation of a Nation Through Real Parenting *Perform the Most Important Task of All—Raising Your Children*	929-6	9.95
Mommy Says *292 Helpful Hints for Moms...and Dads Too!*	961-10	6.95
1001 Things We Would Have Told Our Kids *Had They Ever Listened*	989-10	6.95
Talking Justice *602 Ways To Build & Promote Racial Harmony*	982-2	6.95

ORDER ANY 4 TITLES & GET ONE FREE—PLUS FREE POSTAGE!

Please rush me the following books. I want to save by ordering four books and receive a free book plus free postage. Orders under four books please include $3.00 shipping. CA residents add 8.25% tax.

YOUR ORDER

ORDER #	QUANTITY	UNIT PRICE	TOTAL PRICE

PAYMENT METHOD

❑ Enclosed Check or Money Order

❑ Master Card

❑ Visa

Card Expires _____

Signature _____

RUSH SHIPMENT TO:

(Please print)

Name _____

Organization _____

Address _____

City/State/Zip _____

R & E Publishers ● P.O. Box 2008 ● Saratoga, CA 95070
● (408) 866-6303 ● FAX (408) 866-0825